IS
BREAST
BEST?

HAMLYN HELP YOURSELF GUIDE

IS BREAST BEST?

NICKY ADAMSON

HAMLYN

First published in 1990 by
The Hamlyn Publishing Goup Limited
a division of the Octopus Publishing Group
Michelin House, 81 Fulham Road,
London SW3 6RB

ISBN 0 600 57071 1

Illustrations by Pat Ludlow
Typeset by Dorchester Typesetting Group Ltd
Printed and bound in Great Britain by
Collins, Glasgow

Contents

Introduction   **7**

1 Thinking about feeding   **9**
Feeding, growth and development · Protection
against disease · Feeding and allergies · Feeding
and caring · Practical considerations · Making the
choice

2 How breast feeding works   **24**
Structure of the breasts · How milk is produced

3 Starting to breast feed   **32**
After the birth · Feeding in the first few days · How
to feed · Length and timing of feeds · Winding ·
When your milk comes in · Comfortable positions
for breast feeding

4 Problem solving   **46**
How fathers can help · Getting advice · Enough
milk · Weight loss and gain · Sore nipples ·
Cracked nipples · Leaking · Blocked ducts · Mastitis ·
Breast abscess · Problems with let-down · The
sleepy baby · The resistant baby

5 Some special circumstances   **63**
After a Caesarean · Breast feeding twins ·
Expressing milk · The jaundiced baby · Babies in
special care · Problems with metabolism ·
Premature babies · Physically and mentally
handicapped babies · After a stillbirth

6 Breast feeding and family life   **80**
Looking after yourself · Getting enough rest · Your diet · Fathers and breast feeding · Feeding and sleeping · Feeding and crying · 'Colic' · If you feel depressed · Resuming love-making · Breast feeding and fertility · The active mother · Getting out and about · Going back to work · Changing from breast to bottle · Brothers and sisters

7 Bottle feeding   **100**
Equipment for bottle feeding · Bottles and teats · Sterilizing equipment · How to sterilize · Sterilizing in a hurry · Formula milk · Making up feeds · How much milk · Giving a feed · Winding

8 Weaning   **112**
Introducing solid food · Giving solid food · Your baby's diet · Drinking from a cup · Self-feeding · Breast feeding the older baby

9 Looking after your breasts   **120**
Breast self-examination · What to report to your doctor

Useful addresses   **125**

Introduction

Feeding a baby is basic to parenthood and breast feeding is the most natural method. There is something extremely moving about the sight of a small baby suckling contentedly, eyes closed or perhaps gazing adoringly into the eyes of the person feeding him, maybe gripping an adult finger with a small hand and with toes curling and uncurling with undisguised pleasure. A baby's instinct to feed is incredibly strong, not surprisingly since it is literally a life and death matter for him. Yet it is odd how something so natural and fundamental as infant feeding causes so much anxiety to parents and so much debate among professionals.

Perhaps it is because people want to do the best for their babies that feeding does seem something of a minefield, especially for first time parents. Many people don't think twice about it – for them breast is best and no discussion is needed. For others it may not seem so obvious: perhaps they haven't had any close experience of breast feeding mothers, or they may have anxieties about their ability to feed their babies. Even the most convinced couple may come up against unforeseen problems for which they need to be prepared. So rather than having a last minute panic just as the baby is about to be born, or risking the confusion of conflicting advice when faced with feeding difficulties after the birth, it is worth using the time you have during pregnancy to weigh up the pros and cons, and with the help of this book and the advice of experienced friends and professionals, come to an informed choice together.

The following chapters are there to assist you, first to find out why breast feeding is the most natural way to feed your baby, and then to help mothers to achieve successful and relaxed breast feeding. It doesn't ignore the parents who prefer to bottle feed their babies or change to bottle feeding before their babies are fully weaned on to solid food. The emphasis is on contented and fulfilled parents and babies for whom feeding is a mutually happy experience.

ONE

Thinking about feeding

The simple answer to the question 'Is Breast Best?' is, of course, yes. However, like most aspects of parenting, the subject of infant feeding is not as simple as it should be because so many factors can influence your decision. In the years following the Second World War there was a strong move away from breast feeding towards bottle feeding in the western world. Up to the mid-sixties only about 25 per cent of babies were breast fed, and the majority of people now in their twenties or thirties would have been bottle fed. Many people may never see a baby being breast fed until they start to come into contact with mothers of their own age who opt to breast feed. In the past it was felt that bottle feeding allowed parents more control over exactly how much milk their babies were getting, and that weight gain, which was seen as one of the major indicators that babies were growing 'properly', could be monitored more closely. There was also much more emphasis on getting a baby into a 'routine' of strict four-hourly feeds, which the mechanics of bottle feeding suited much better.

However, there has been a welcome shift away from those rather draconian rules about routines and schedules. Many older women may remember the misery of listening to their babies crying piteously but being advised not to go and pick them up to avoid 'spoiling' them because it wasn't 'time for a feed' or 'the baby's got to learn'. It is now known that feeding means a lot more than just nutrition and that whether you use breast or bottle, it is of positive benefit for you to follow your own instincts about picking up your baby when he cries, whether he's hungry or not.

You may well be asked by the doctor or midwife at your first antenatal check-up whether you are going to feed by breast or bottle. This is just one of the routine questions that are asked of all mothers. It gives a rounded view of them to everyone looking after them during their pregnancy and after the birth. Nowadays you will be encouraged to opt for breast feeding. However, don't feel you have to give a definitive answer if you haven't made up your mind; just say you haven't decided yet. Even if you have made up your mind one way or another at this early stage of your pregnancy, you can always change your mind later. Don't feel you have to stick to what you said six months ago if after the birth you want to do something different. It is your choice, and people's moods and circumstances change, especially during the highly charged and emotional experience of pregnancy and birth. The midwives and doctors will not think badly of you – they only want to know so that they can advise and help you if need be.

During your pregnancy there will probably be antenatal preparation classes which you can attend at the hospital or perhaps a local health centre which will include infant feeding among the topics. You could also get in touch with one of the independent groups such as the National Childbirth Trust, La Leche League or the Association of Breastfeeding Mothers which run courses or support groups locally, usually in the informal setting of another mother's home. Either way it helps to attend classes or join one of these organizations because you will meet other expectant parents in your own area; some may be first-timers, others more experienced. It is extremely helpful to discuss feeding with a mother who has gone through it all once or twice before, and to trade ideas among yourselves. At the end of the day, however, the decision is yours.

Feeding, growth and development

All mothers have the capacity to breast feed their own babies. Breast feeding is after all only the final phase of the process of nurturing a new human being that occurs throughout your pregnancy. The job which was being done by the placenta is just transferred to the breasts after the birth of your baby. It follows that the milk which is produced by the breasts is perfectly suited to the needs of your baby, just as the nutrients being passed across to the baby via the placenta and umbilical cord were exactly right for the growing fetus in the uterus.

In the natural world, all mammals feed their young on their own milk – it is one of the essential biological factors which binds together species as diverse as elephants, mice, wolves and whales. Just as all these species are completely different, so too is the composition of the milk that is produced to meet the differing needs of their young. This is exactly the same for human beings and cows – human milk is tailored specifically for human infants, while cow's milk is designed for calves.

Human milk contains everything a baby needs to be completely satisfied. It has exactly the right balance of proteins, fats and carbohydrates which can be fully absorbed by the baby with very little waste. By contrast, in its natural state, cow's milk has a higher protein content, particularly of the casein type, which is hard for babies to digest, and lower carbohydrate (lactose) levels.

Casein is needed for the building of body tissue. It is not surprising that cow's milk contains about three times more than human milk when you compare the size of a calf at birth in proportion to its mother with that of a human baby. A calf is a herd animal; like horses, sheep and deer, the species has evolved so that the young can be up on their feet and within the protective circle of the herd if necessary within a few hours of the birth. Muscle and bone development are of prime importance whereas for human infants the growth and development of the brain and nerve pathways are paramount. As a result the amount of body building proteins is proportionately less in breast milk, and those nutrients required for brain growth, especially lactose, are more.

Babies need fat to build up a warm layer of insulation against heat loss while their internal temperature control is still immature. They also need it to provide the high energy levels necessary for fast growth. A baby grows proportionately more in the first six months than at any other time of his life. In fact, the fat content of cow's milk is about the same as that in human milk, but is absorbed much less efficiently than the fat in human milk, and is therefore wasted. It can also lead to babies becoming overweight.

Another difference between cow's milk in its natural state and human breast milk is the higher salt and phosphate contents. This puts a burden on the baby's immature kidneys which have to work very hard to eliminate the unwanted sodium, this means that they also lose water which could lead to dangerous dehydration. Although there is more iron by volume in cow's milk, once again it is in a form less easily absorbed than in breast milk, and could provoke intestinal bleeding.

Of course, all the marked differences outlined here are between breast milk and cow's milk as it comes to you on the doorstep or on the supermarket shelf. No one would now dream of giving a baby under six months or even older a bottle of ordinary milk. The manufacturers of infant formulae, whether in powdered or liquid form, have worked hard to modify the cow's milk on which it is based as far as possible to mimic breast milk. They have included all the necessary vitamins and minerals in the right proportions to make it as safe and nutritious as possible. They have reduced the salt content, added iron and other vitamins and minerals in a safe form, reduced protein levels and changed its nature to make it easier to digest, and adjusted the fat content. There is no doubt that infant formulae nowadays do provide a very acceptable alternative food for babies, on which they thrive, but there is no denying the fact that they are not the same as breast milk, which has many other properties which an artificial formula can never have.

Protection against disease

Research over the last twenty years has discovered that breast milk has a very important function in protecting the young baby from disease. During pregnancy, antibodies from the mother pass across the placenta into the baby's bloodstream and these help to ward off certain infections which would be dangerous while the immune system is immature. These remain in the baby's bloodstream for some time after the birth which is why your baby's programme of immunization starts at least three months after birth, and sometimes much more. (A notable exception to this is whooping cough, whose antibodies are too big to cross the placenta, which is why fairly early immunization is essential against this dangerous disease.)

This process of maternal protection continues with breast feeding. Colostrum, the name given to the creamy substance which is produced by the breasts in the first few days after birth (see p. 35) is particularly important in this. It actually contains the same living white cells called leucocytes which are the first line of defence in fighting infectious bacteria and viruses. The colostrum is particularly rich in these in the first few hours after birth (see p. 32).

It used to be thought that breast feeding for a few days after the birth was enough to give a baby protection from infection by at least exposing him to the helpful colostrum. In western societies with their high standards of health and hygiene generally, it was considered that the switch to bottle feeding at this point would not make any appreciable difference to a baby's risk of infection. In many parts of the world where water supplies are suspect, and general standards of hygiene lower, bottle feeding is actively discouraged. Bacterial infections causing dangerous gastrointestinal illnesses are more likely to occur when it is difficult to maintain the sterile conditions necessary for safe bottle feeding. By contrast, breast milk is automatically clean and the milk itself has been found to help protect against these types of infection, and against respiratory diseases.

It is only recently that research has shown that the same principles apply in the West, particularly if feeding is maintained for at least three calendar months (thirteen weeks). Doctors in Scotland have found that babies breast fed for at least this time suffered significantly less from serious gastrointestinal illness requiring hospitalization than bottle fed babies, not just during the time they were being breast fed, but up to the age of twelve months. This is a most important finding; it means that the longer you go on breast feeding, the longer your baby is effectively protected against infection, especially vomiting and diarrhoea, and to a lesser extent, respiratory diseases. It is worth emphasizing that gastrointestinal illnesses can be dangerous for any child and particularly for young babies who rapidly dehydrate. Extreme cases require hospitalization with the attendant distress for the baby and worry and disruption for the parents.

Feeding and allergies

Apart from the proven protection against infection, it is thought that breast fed babies are less likely to suffer from allergies later in childhood. This is a fairly controversial area, because there is so much research still to be done into the nature and causes of allergies generally, but if there is a history of allergic reaction in the families of either parent, resulting in conditions such as eczema, asthma or hay fever, then you will probably be advised to breast feed if possible. There is enough evidence to suggest that even if it doesn't prevent allergies completely, breast feeding does seem to reduce the severity of this particular type of allergic reaction.

A very few babies are found to be allergic to the protein in cow's milk itself. The first signs of this may be diarrhoea, which could be blood stained, and for which no other cause can be diagnosed. In extreme cases cow's milk allergy can result in swelling of the mouth and throat which interferes with feeding and breathing and results in a very distressed baby. This form of reaction has become very uncommon since modern methods have enabled the protein in infant formula to be modified to a great extent. However, cases do still occur, but can be treated by removing cow's milk from the diet for six to twelve months after which there is usually no longer a problem. Cow's milk allergy should always be treated by a doctor. Allergy is a complex subject and it is dangerous to ascribe any problem with a young baby to 'allergy' without a definite diagnosis (see p. 85).

Feeding and caring

There has been a tendency in recent years for those campaigning for a general return to breast feeding to emphasize the beneficial psychological aspects when compared with bottle feeding. They point to the special relationship which is built up between the mother and her breast-fed baby especially if feeding is begun immediately after the birth. There is much truth in this for the mothers who have no difficulty in establishing breast feeding, whose birth experience has been relatively trouble-free and who have had no prior anxieties about feeding in particular and parenting in general. For the majority of women who breast feed it is wonderfully relaxing and pleasurable in its own right, just as it is for the baby, and it becomes part and parcel of the love which they build between them.

However, this isn't the case for every woman. The very success of the campaign for breast feeding may instil unforeseen feelings of guilt in some women who either can't or don't want to breast feed, especially straight after the birth. Some may feel that they won't be giving their babies enough love and close contact if they bottle feed and so embark on breast feeding from a sense of duty rather than anything else. If breast feeding proves difficult to establish, and in those circumstances, it might well do so (see p. 57), the mother may turn to bottle feeding but at the same time feel she has failed her baby, which is a very unfortunate way to start a relationship with a newborn. Equally, if a woman simply doesn't want to feed her baby in that way, she shouldn't be made to feel guilty, because the baby still gets closeness and cuddles at feeding times if the feeds are given from the bottle.

There are benefits on both sides. Bottle feeding can be done by either parent, and the closeness of the bond from the physical act of feeding can be developed equally by mother and father – or any other caring person for that matter. Babies soon learn to recognize the bottle and respond to it favourably just as they do to the breast. Yet it undoubtedly is more impersonal; it is much easier for a baby to suck a bottle teat so the period spent feeding will generally be shorter, and the time spent cuddling and generally handling the baby is likely to be less overall. Breast fed babies feed at their own pace and although at times breast feeding mothers may occasionally find this frustrating if they want to get to the shops before they shut or fetch an older child from school, this 'pacing' is thought to influence positively a baby's normal emotional and physical development.

The old school of thought believed that too much handling and picking up of a baby was bad for him in that he would become spoilt and 'too dependent' on his parents. How he was supposed to be anything else has never been satisfactorily explained! Fortunately this harsh regime has fallen into disrepute, and on the whole it has been found that breast fed babies are more independent and less clingy at twelve months and later when they begin to socialize than their bottle fed counterparts. Obviously this is a simplification since so many psychological and environmental factors have to be taken into account when assessing a child's personality, but it does seem that breast feeding is one of them. In addition it does no harm for a mother to slow down to the rhythm of breast feeding and not to worry so much about domestic chores (see p. 82).

Another psychological factor which may affect mothers' decisions about breast feeding is the attitude of their partners. For many parents embarking on pregnancy, birth and baby care for the first time this can be a crucial area of influence. Most fathers these days are as interested and involved as their partners in their offsprings' development as much before the birth as after it. This is usually encouraged in antenatal care by inviting both partners to clinic visits, allowing fathers to be present during ultrasound scans and, especially, assuming that they will be there to support their partners through labour and witness the birth of their babies. Fathers are also welcome at antenatal classes – even when they take place normally in the daytime, at least one evening get-together is usually arranged to enable working fathers to attend.

Even so, when the moment arrives, a few fathers may still feel ambivalent about breast feeding. After all, until that time they have seen their partners' breasts in a very different light – in terms of sex, and this view will have been rein-

17

forced by images of women in the media all round them. Indeed, many younger women who find breast feeding distasteful probably do·so because they are still confused about this dual role for their breasts.

Fathers can add to this confusion by objecting to their partners' breasts being 'exposed' during feeding, especially to other men. Again this is unnecessary since breast feeding does not mean having to strip to the waist or flaunt your body to the world – far from it. A father may even be rather jealous of the breast feeding baby, although he may not like to admit it. If he feels at all excluded, and a baby can seem to take up an awful lot of a mother's attention, he may transmit his annoyance to his partner, causing her directly or indirectly to change to bottle feeding instead.

This is a pity, for it needn't be like that. If you can discuss the pros and cons of feeding methods together, or even better within a group of other expectant parents, both partners can work through any misgivings they may have about either method. Some fathers favour bottle feeding because they want to have an equal share in the nurturing of their babies and feel that breast feeding puts an unfair burden on their partners. However, a father can have an equal role in parenting the breast fed baby by providing the infra-structure within the home to make breast feeding simple and straightforward, especially in the early weeks. Watching a baby at the breast of the person with whom you have decided to share your life is an extremely happy experience for fathers, especially when you know that it is the best nourishment that your baby can have. There is plenty of time for paternal cuddling when the feed is over.

There are however some women who actually can't breast feed, and some babies for whom bottles are a better option. An adopted baby obviously has to be bottle fed as this is what he will be used to by the time he comes to the adoptive parents – even a newborn isn't released to the parents until six weeks of age in the U.K. (Lactation can be stimulated if the adopted baby is practically newborn, but this is very rare.) If a mother suffers from a chronic condition requiring certain types of medication regularly, it could be a problem since minute quantities of the medication can pass across to the baby through the milk, and may not be good for him. In this case bottle feeding is safer and at least you know that for once this is best for your baby. If your baby has a general allergy to lactose, whether from cow's or human milk then obviously a non-milk substitute has to be given by bottle. Again this is a very rare condition.

It may be that because you are going back to work very soon after the birth or have other pressing commitments, you think that it will simply be easier to start as you mean to go on, with the bottle. Many health care professionals try to persuade women to breast feed even for a few days to provide their babies with the protection from infection found in colostrum. While this is a sensible precaution, a mother who wants to bottle feed from the start shouldn't feel guilty.

However, if you think your professional commitments are going to make it difficult for you to breast feed perhaps because you work irregular shifts or your job takes you away a lot, think carefully before you decide to go exclusively for bottle feeding. The dedicated mother can express milk successfully to maintain the supply even when she is away, and if you have time to establish feeding after the birth, it may be that you can get into a routine of one or two breast feeds per day only. However, this does require a lot of motivation and if you are worrying about it you are likely to impede your milk supply anyway, so it is probably better to bottle feed and know that both you and your baby are going to be more content.

There are women who simply find the whole idea of breast feeding distasteful. This can be for a number of reasons: some younger mothers of first-time babies may still be coming to terms with their own sexuality, let alone the responsibilities of parenthood. Bottle feeding is one way of holding the whole business of baby care literally at arm's length. Other mothers dislike the idea of being at a baby's beck and call, of being 'cow-like'. They feel it restricts their freedom of movement in that society as a whole still frowns on mothers feeding their babies in public places. Many women also feel embarrassed about the idea of breast feeding, particularly in front of other people. If they feel they have to hide away every time they want to feed their babies it is no wonder that either they don't start at all or eventually give up to avoid being stuck at home all the time.

While mothers should perhaps think about the impact on people around them when they need to breast feed while out, and remember that old attitudes are quite difficult to eradicate, it is perfectly possible to breast feed so discreetly that even the most censorious person won't notice (see p. 94)! In addition, it is worth campaigning for more large stores, cafes, transport waiting areas and local authority amenities to provide quiet places where a mother can breast feed and if necessary change her baby in comfort. With the wider acceptance of breast feeding again this may soon cease to be an issue. It is to be hoped that girls, and boys, will increasingly be taking breast feeding for granted either by seeing their own younger siblings or cousins being breast fed, or learning about it at school as a matter of course.

At the end of the day, however, whatever your reasons for opting for the bottle rather than the breast, it is important to emphasize that millions of babies who have been bottle fed from birth are just as well-loved and cared for as their breast fed counterparts, and develop quite normally.

Practical considerations

Although it is sensible to concentrate first and foremost on the health and developmental aspects of breast feeding and bottle feeding, there are some more practical considerations which provide back-up in helping parents to choose. Breast feeding is undoubtedly both cheaper and more convenient than bottle feeding. Breast milk is available at any time of the day or night. It needs no preparation and is always completely satisfying. Contrary to what some people think, it is impossible to 'empty' the breasts. Milk will continue to be made as long as the baby stimulates them by sucking (see p. 31).

Of course, only the mother can feed the baby, although you can express milk to be fed in a bottle by someone else if necessary. Particularly in the first three months when feeds are frequent, it really does save time and effort, especially at night, to know that your baby can be pacified without any forethought required. Experienced mothers know that forethought is a commodity in short supply in the first few months of new motherhood! By contrast, bottles need to be made up ahead of time, and even if you use the convenient (but expensive) ready-made liquid formulae, you still need to maintain the strictest hygiene. If you are caught short and have to make up a feed in a hurry, bottles have a nasty habit of being too hot just at the moment when you have a hungry baby bawling for food, *now* . . .

Breast feeding costs nothing. Most people on a normal healthy diet do not have to spend any more on food than at other times (see p. 84). The only extra expense which mothers may have is the purchase of breast pads and nursing bras which are helpful (though not essential) for the first few months. If you bottle feed, however, apart from the initial expense of bottles, teats and sterilizing equipment, there is also a significant weekly outlay on infant formula. This is an aspect of the whole debate which is sometimes not emphasized enough, particularly with lower income families, although some help in the form of milk tokens is available to families on income support. In addition, if you wean from breast to bottle after breast feeding has been established for a while, you may find that you have to experiment with different types of bottles and teats, which adds to the expense.

Breast-fed babies produce less offensive stools because their bodies absorb the milk more efficiently so there is less waste. By contrast babies fed on infant formula have quite smelly nappies since they do not absorb as much of the solids in cow's milk and it has to be got rid of. This may seem a trivial point, but it is quite significant in that a breast fed baby may have fewer dirty nappies which means less washing and, more importantly, less chance of the nappy rash associated with dirty nappies (see p. 87). It is fair to say however that breast and bottle fed babies wet their nappies equally, so there is no difference in the frequency of nappy changes overall!

Finally, breast feeding does have a physiological impact on the mother herself. Breast feeding in the hours and days immediately following the birth helps the uterus to contract properly (see p. 33), lessening the chance of dangerous haemorrhage or infection. It also uses up special layers of fat laid down in your body during pregnancy, and helps you to regain your figure more quickly. Some women find that they actually lose weight and become slimmer than before they were pregnant. On the other hand, it often also has the effect of reducing the size of your breasts. This may appear to be an advantage to some women, but to others – and their partners – it is less welcome!

Making the choice

For some couples approaching the whole business of pregnancy and baby care, the added pressure of deciding about feeding may be something they could do without. Yet feeding is so vital that nobody should grudge it a little time and thought. You will undoubtedly be encouraged to breast feed by those caring for you during your pregnancy, while on the other hand your friends or family might be saying something different. If you have made up your mind, that's fine; if not it is hoped that this chapter has helped to put the arguments across. It is worth bearing in mind the proud boast of one president of an American infant formula manufacturer, quoted in one of the La Leche League's books: 'Our product is second best to breast.'

TWO

How breast feeding works

Breast feeding can begin as soon as your baby is born; you yourself don't have to do anything special as it is an automatic process triggered by the level of various hormones in your body. Under the control of a small area of the brain called the hypothalamus, the pituitary gland at the base of the brain secretes the hormones which prepared your body for childbearing and brought about the changes necessary to sustain the pregnancy. These are also working to prepare your breasts for the final link in the chain – feeding your baby after the birth.

Structure of the breasts

Breasts vary enormously in size, but all are essentially constructed the same way. Breasts do not have muscles, they are naturally supported by the pectoral muscles around them. (If you stand in front of a mirror holding each wrist with the opposite hand and push firmly outward towards each elbow you will see your breasts being lifted by the tensing of the chest muscles.) Instead breasts mainly consist of fatty tissue – the bigger the breasts the higher proportion of fat there is in them. Having small breasts does not mean that you are less able to breast feed; on the contrary, small breasts produce milk very efficiently while large or

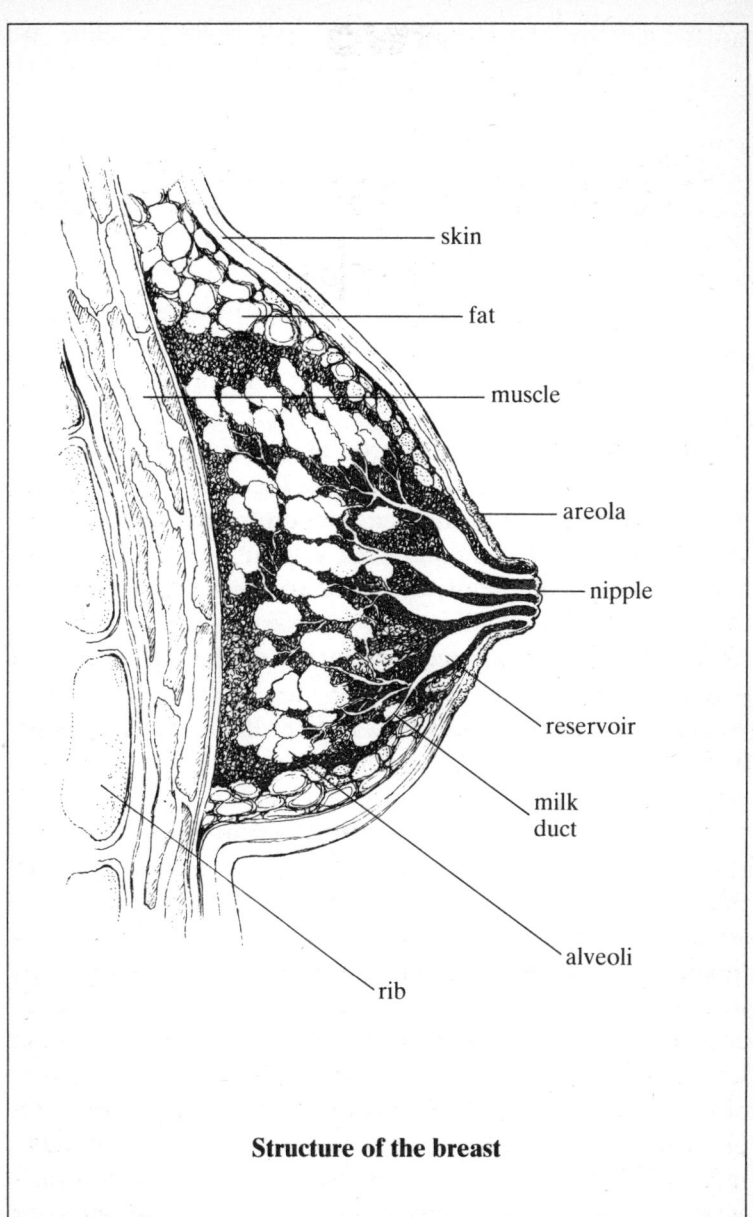

skin

fat

muscle

areola

nipple

reservoir

milk
duct

alveoli

rib

Structure of the breast

pendulous breasts sometimes impede breast feeding by making it difficult for the baby to grasp the nipple properly (see p. 37).

Within this fatty tissue are millions of milk-producing cells lining the inside of tiny sacs called alveoli. The milk-producing cells are in turn surrounded by tiny muscle cells (called myoepithelial cells) which squeeze the milk into the ducts. There are about eighteen segments in the breast each of which has a main milk duct leading towards the nipple, and the milk produced in each group of alveoli drains into a particular duct. Each of the eighteen milk ducts ends with an opening at the nipple, and they balloon slightly behind the nipple so that a little milk can form a reservoir there. The nipple itself is made up of erectile tissue; you will probably have noticed that stimulation – whether by touch, sexual excitement or simply when exposed to cold temperatures – will make your normally soft nipple much more rigid. The nipple has lots of tiny openings, one for each milk duct, and it is surrounded by a circle of similarly coloured skin called the areola.

Just as the ovaries and uterus are prepared for reproduction, so the breasts of all young women grow and are prepared for infant feeding during adolescence. Although the openings in the nipple are practically invisible, they are there, and even if you do not realize it so are the alveoli and other structures inside the breast. During pregnancy, however, the action of the hormone oestrogen causes an enormous increase in the number of alveoli. This process begins almost at once; in fact lots of women find that they are experiencing changes in their breasts before they have even confirmed that they are pregnant.

The breasts temporarily increase in size during pregnancy and may feel tender, for instance while running or riding, and can make love-making a bit uncomfortable. (Pregnancy generally requires a rethink of regular love-making positions.) You'll find it more comfortable if you wear a good supporting bra during the day. If you need to buy new ones in a bigger size and you have definitely decided to breast feed, it makes sense to buy nursing bras with flaps or hooks to avoid paying out again after the birth.

Oestrogen also causes changes to the areola and nipple. Their colour darkens and the nipple elongates slightly, and little protuberances, called Montgomery's tubercles, become much more pronounced on the areola. It is thought that these aid the natural lubrication of the nipple, helping to keep it supple during breast feeding and avoiding the danger of cracks forming in the skin (see p. 52).

During the latter part of pregnancy you may notice that your nipples start secreting a creamy substance, which may form slight crusts as it dries. This is colostrum, the liquid that precedes the true milk which doesn't start being produced properly until a few days after the birth. There is absolutely no need to express colostrum during pregnancy; it won't make any difference to milk production after the birth which happens automatically (see p. 30). If you notice deposits of dried colostrum, simply wipe them away gently with a face flannel or sponge when you are having a bath.

Care of the breasts during pregnancy

You do not have to do anything special to your breasts or nipples during pregnancy to prepare them for breast feeding. Your breasts will become larger and may feel slightly lumpy, but this is generally nothing to worry about and is simply a sign that the hormones are doing their work in increasing the number of alveoli in the breast. If you are at all worried, however, discuss it with your doctor or midwife.

Periodically during your antenatal check-ups the midwife or doctor will examine your breasts and check that the nipples stand out sufficiently on stimulation. Just as the size of your breasts makes no difference to successful breast feeding, so the size of your nipples isn't important either as long as they protrude a little. As will be seen later (see p. 35), the nipple itself is not as important as the areola in actually delivering milk into the baby's mouth, this will happen if the baby is latched on to the breast properly.

If your nipples are quite flat your midwife may suggest gently rolling them between your fingers occasionally during pregnancy to encourage them to stand out, but even this is simply to reassure you. So long as they do stand out there is no need to make an issue of it. You can also try an exercise called the Hoffman Technique, which consists of placing your index fingers on the skin either side of the areola and gently stretching the skin horizontally, then doing the same manoeuvre vertically. If your nipples are actually inverted – which is a much rarer condition than is sometimes made out – you may be given a breast shield to wear inside your bra to encourage the nipple to protrude.

For most women however, no such exercises or devices are necessary. There is no need to scrub your nipples vigorously or use creams or sprays to 'toughen' them, in fact this is positively bad. The skin of the nipples is naturally tough but also very supple; anything which has the effect of drying out the natural oils is more likely to result in soreness and cracking when your baby eventually starts to suckle (see p. 52).

How milk is produced

Once your baby is born and the placenta is no longer producing oestrogen, the levels of prolactin, the hormone that stimulates milk production, rise sharply and the cells in the breast start producing milk. This happens even with premature births (see p. 75).

Although milk starts being produced after the birth, it only comes in properly after two or three days. Before that the breasts feel quite soft and continue to produce colostrum. Gradually milk starts to come in so that there is a mixture of colostrum and milk, and the colostrum content reduces until milk only is being produced. You will soon realize when the milk comes in properly, because your breasts swell with the greatly increased blood supply and the milk itself, and they may feel engorged. This is the time when frequent feeding is essential both for your own comfort and for the successful establishment of breast feeding.

Milk will only continue to be produced at this point and indeed at any time during babyhood, if stimulated by the baby at the breast. Human breasts do not store large quantities of milk like cow's udders – in this respect we are most 'un-cow-like' – since milk production is linked directly to the needs of the baby. When the baby sucks at the nipple the nerve endings there send messages to the brain which are then transmitted to the pituitary gland in order to make it produce more prolactin. The higher levels of prolactin in the bloodstream in turn stimulate the milk-producing cells in the breast to produce more milk. The more the baby suckles, the more milk will be produced, which is why frequent feeds when your baby asks for them are so important (see p. 38).

When milk is produced it fills the tiny sacs of the alveoli, but it does not simply trickle down the milk ducts towards the nipple. Instead the tiny muscles surrounding the milk-producing cells contract and squeeze the milk down. This action is under the control of another hormone, oxytocin, which is also stimulated by the baby sucking on the nipple, and is known as the 'let-down reflex'. Some women feel a characteristic tingling or gentle prickling feeling inside their breasts at the start of a feed, others don't feel anything. However, a little milk usually leaks from the nipple which lets you know that the milk is there. Generally speaking you will only feel this at the start of a feed. This doesn't mean there is only one let-down per feed, on the contrary, once

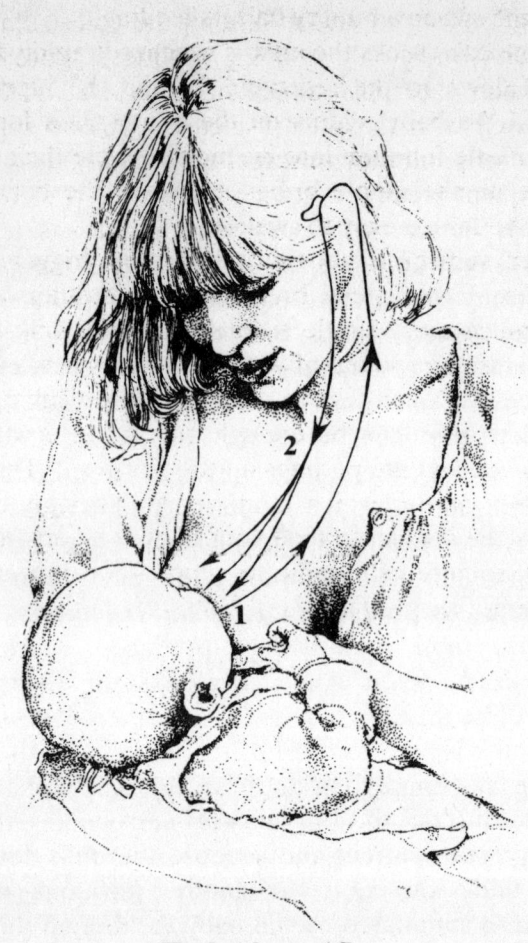

The let-down reflex

1   When the baby sucks, nerves in the areola send messages to the hypothalamus in the brain.
2   The hypothalamus signals the pituitary gland to release oxytocin which causes the muscle cells of the alveoli to squeeze milk down to the ducts to the nipple.

feeding is established, milk can come down as often as seven or eight times when a hungry baby is feeding.

When the baby sucks the milk is squeezed rapidly into the ducts and down to the reservoirs behind the nipple. The pressure of the baby's gums on the areola then forces the milk like a little fountain into his mouth, while the action of his tongue on the nipple brings it well to the back of his mouth so the milk is easy to swallow.

However, sucking is not the only way to trigger the let-down reflex. Experienced breast feeding mothers can tell you that much more subtle signals can bring milk literally flooding down. The sound of your baby's cry – and even that of someone else's baby – can do it, and just thinking about feeding your baby can be enough, for instance when you have been out and are perhaps a little late back. This reflex is a complex matter which is influenced strongly by your emotions – the instinct to feed your baby is a very deep one – but it is equally vulnerable to suppression if you've got any problems (see p. 57).

THREE

Starting to breast feed

After the birth

The best time to start breast feeding is as soon as possible after the birth. Babies are born with a very strong sucking reflex. It has been shown that they make sucking movements inside the uterus and some babies even suck their thumbs or fingers when their limb movements bring their hands into contact with their faces. Putting the baby to the breast when you first hold him is probably one of the most amazing and yet practical things you can do at this stage – amazing because your brand new baby is responding to you as a mother by suckling immediately, and practical because it is the natural first step in getting breast feeding established quickly.

Unless you have had to have quite a lot of pain-killing drugs during your labour your baby will be very alert at this point. Many people are surprised by this, but it is a fact that after a normal delivery babies will be awake for at least an hour after the birth, and are able to focus on the face of someone near them. When you hold the baby in your arms to breast feed you are just the right distance away for him to see you and you will discover that your new baby really is looking at you.

You may not feel very expert at feeding at this moment – you won't feel any let-down because your milk has not come in – but you and your baby will be making a start on an important learning process. Your baby won't know exactly where the breast is, but has another important reflex, called the rooting response. If you gently stroke his cheek he will automatically turn towards it and search for the nipple. At this stage he'll probably need a little gentle guidance with the helping hand of your partner or a midwife supporting his head, but he'll manage.

This early feed has a number of benefits. It helps to get lactation under way as soon as possible by stimulating the whole process of hormonal change. In addition, the release of the hormone oxytocin doesn't only effect the muscle cells in the breast (see p. 29), but also those of the uterus, causing it to contract. You will probably feel cramping after-pains, like severe period pains, at the time and for a few days after the birth whenever you breast feed, which could be accompanied by a certain amount of vaginal bleeding. This is perfectly normal and in fact a very good thing, since it is helping the uterus to return to its usual non-pregnant size quickly and with less likelihood of serious bleeding or infection. It also helps of course to bring you and your baby close together right from the start.

Obviously if your baby is born by Caesarean section under general anaesthetic you will not be able to breast feed immediately (see p. 64). In this case it is not going to do you or your baby any harm to start breast feeding a little later. The same applies if your baby is a little distressed and requires some attention immediately after the birth. Although this may cause you some anxiety at the time it is reassuring when at last you are able to hold your baby to put him to the breast at that point.

If you have a Caesarean under an epidural anaesthetic, which means that you are awake but don't feel any pain, you can still put your baby to the breast if he is well by asking the midwife to lay him on the bed beside you (see p. 64). You may alternatively have had a difficult or long, tiring labour and may just feel like turning over and going to sleep when it's all over. Again, you or your partner could ask the midwife to let the baby lie beside you to suckle for a time while you drowse. It doesn't require any effort on your part but you will both benefit from it.

You may find that some midwives are reluctant to allow you to have your baby in the bed with you to feed lying down in this way. However, if your partner is with you he can sit beside you to reassure the midwife that the baby is not going to roll off the bed.

Feeding in the first few days

Whether you are able to feed immediately after the birth of your baby or not, the serious business of getting breast feeding established will begin when you and your baby are together during the first couple of days after the birth. Unless you had a home birth or a so-called 'domino' delivery, which means that you will be back at home within six hours of the birth, it will be back on the postnatal ward that this process begins.

Full-term babies have a layer of fat laid down in the last few weeks of pregnancy which provides them with energy while they wait for their mothers' milk to come in. This is why a baby always loses some weight in the first day or so, but will usually have regained his birth weight by the time he is about ten days old. So even if you are very tired and need a good long sleep after the birth, there is no need for the baby to be given a bottle even if it is only water. Let the midwives on the ward know that you would prefer them not to do this; in fact this may be a job for your partner if you have already gone to sleep.

If necessary ask the midwives to wake you if your baby is crying, this is not usually necessary, especially when your baby is in a cot beside your bed. If you aren't particularly tired, or only need a short rest, you can pick your baby up to nurse whenever you feel both you and he are ready.

Newborn babies often sleep for a few hours after the initial. wakeful period and will appreciate a feed when they wake up, which is helpful when you are both going through this early learning process as he will be keen to suckle.

As has already been explained, at first your breasts only produce colostrum, the creamy substance which is full of protective antibodies. Colostrum is high in protein, and low in fat and carbohydrate, so is easier for your baby's immature digestive system to cope with. Your baby is also likely to sleep longer between feeds; as mature milk starts to come in feeds become more frequent.

At this stage your breasts will still be quite soft and manageable, with none of the discomfort sometimes associated with the arrival of mature milk. This makes these first feeds a lot easier to manage. To feed properly, a baby has to draw the whole nipple into his mouth so that his gums are squeezing the areola, forcing the milk out from the ducts behind it and into the the back of his throat. This is crucial; if the baby only has hold of the nipple he will not get much milk and you will soon become sore, thus setting up a vicious circle of frustration on the one part and pain on the other. If you remember that the whole of the nipple must lie along his tongue you will realize that he had to get hold of the areola to enable this to happen.

Although you should get into the habit of washing your hands before a feed, there is no need to wash your breasts immediately beforehand. They will be quite clean enough from regular bathing. It is best not to use any special creams or sprays, since the latter especially dry your skin making soreness and cracking more, not less, likely. They also mask the natural smell of your skin and of the milk. It has been proved that babies can recognize their mothers' particular smell within a few days of the birth and the smell of the milk also attracts them to the breast, so it is best not to wash this away or mask it with chemicals.

How to feed

The best way to explain how to breast feed is to set it out as a few simple steps.

- First of all sit up in bed or on a comfortable chair with arms, well supported by pillows. At this stage a practically upright position is best so you can see what is going on.
- Cradle the baby in your arms so that his head is at the right level for your breast. To make sure that you aren't having to lean forward too much put a pillow across your lap to raise your baby, and have another under the elbow which is supporting your baby's head.
- Turn your baby's whole body slightly so that he is facing you and support his bottom with your hand. His cheek should now be resting against your breast, near the nipple.
- With your free hand, gently tickle his cheek with a finger or your nipple. He will open his mouth and turn towards it.
- Guide the whole nipple into his mouth by lifting it between the forefinger and middle finger just behind the areola. This has the advantage of causing the nipple to protrude. Make sure his gums are grasping the areola and his tongue is under the nipple. He will immediately begin to suck.

At this first proper feed, you will probably have a midwife on hand to advise you and check that the baby is latched on properly. If you aren't sure, ring for the midwife to come and check. In fact your baby will let you know – if he is sucking properly you can see small muscles in his temple moving, and his ears might move as well. He may close his eyes, or alternatively might begin the feeding by gazing fixedly into your face.

If he isn't latched on properly, he may well drop the nipple or just chew on it rather uncomfortably. If this happens remove the nipple from his mouth and start again. You are both going to need practice at getting it right, for

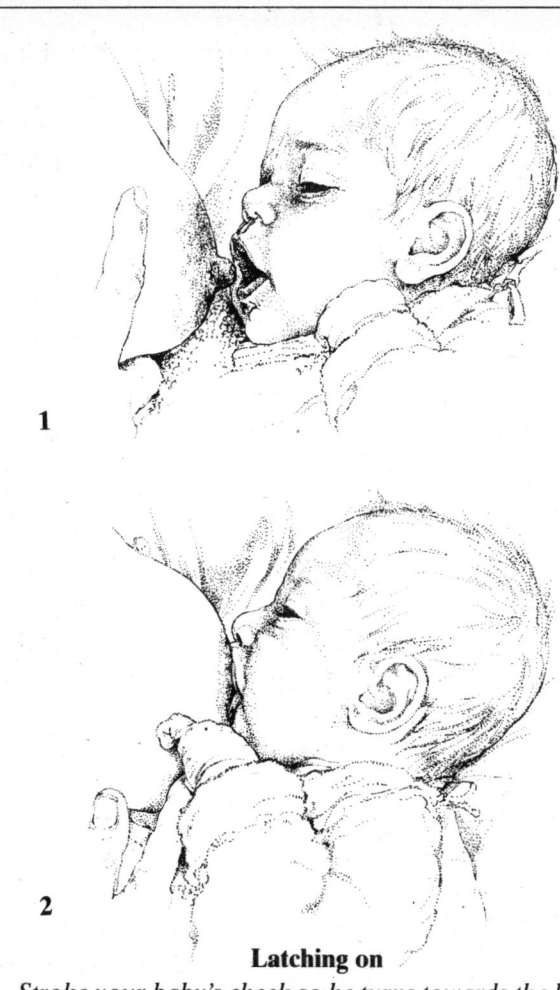

1

2

Latching on

*1   Stroke your baby's cheek so he turns towards the breast
and opens his mouth, then guide your nipple towards him
with your free hand.*

*2   He is latched on properly when his gums are right round
the areola and the whole of the nipple is lying along his
tongue.*

although a baby has the instinct to suck, he still needs to get used to your breasts, and to learn how to obtain milk quickly and efficiently. If he's a bit slow or sleepy, don't force his mouth open, this will just distress him. Just gently guide the nipple towards him against his cheek so he can feel it and smell the milk, and let him take his time in turning towards it. Sometimes expressing a few drops of colostrum or milk on to his lips encourages him to get going.

Length and timing of feeds

Feeding should never be regulated 'by the clock', either in how long your baby stays at the breast or in timing the intervals between feeds. Particularly at this stage babies, and nursing mothers, need frequent feeding. You will probably be given a chart in the hospital on which to enter the times and length of feeds but don't be put off by this. If your baby seems content, the feeds can be as long or as short, and as frequent, as he needs.

In these early days it is important to allow your baby to set the pace. This may mean just a few minutes on each side, or as much as twenty. You may even find that you have forgotten to change over in the middle and your baby has gone to sleep contentedly while feeding only at one breast while you dozed or read a book or talked to your visitors. Again this doesn't matter, although for your own sake it's a good idea to make a note of which breast your baby last suckled so you can switch to the other side next time so you don't become one sided.

Small babies don't feed very fast; you will notice that your baby has bouts of hard sucking interspersed between rests where he simply seems to play with the nipple. This is exactly what he is doing. Babies enjoy the whole sensation of being held and of sucking not just as a source of food but of pleasure and security as well, for these are of course all bound up together in the newborn baby's experience. You will find therefore that sometimes your baby will feed lustily for a few minutes and then release the breast of his own accord, at which point you can change over to the other breast and see if he wants to start again there. On other occasions you may find that as soon as you start to withdraw he will latch on and start sucking vigorously again.

If you do need to change sides, and when your milk starts to come in this is advisable at every feed (see p. 41), don't try simply to pull your nipple out of your baby's mouth if he is still latched on tightly – that is a sure recipe for sore nipples. Instead gently insert your (clean) finger into the corner of his mouth to release the suction, and withdraw your nipple. It is important to take care in doing this in the early stages since sore nipples can be a great disincentive to feeding just at the time you need the greatest motivation.

Winding

Before your milk comes in there is no need to try and bring up wind when you change sides or after a feed as your baby is unlikely to have swallowed much air. Breast fed babies have much less 'wind' than bottle fed ones. Many parents find holding their babies' wobbly heads a bit nerve-racking to start with anyway, so if you think your baby might need winding just hold him gently against your shoulder, supporting the back of his head with your hand. Normally there is no need to do this at all when you change sides, unless your baby obviously doesn't want to feed any more for the moment and you both benefit from a change of position. When you feel a bit more confident about handling him, you can sit him up on your knee gently supporting his head under his chin and very gently rubbing his back. There is no need to rub or bang vigorously.

It is important not to let winding become a big issue in feeding. Anything that makes you anxious can be off-putting at this stage. People may tell you that you must wind the baby between sides and after every feed, but when you have spent three-quarters of an hour feeding at two o'clock in the morning, the last thing you want or need to do is to prolong it for both of you by trying to extract a burp when all either of you really wants to do is to go back to sleep.

When your milk comes in and your baby is gulping it down hungrily you may well find that he does burp when you lift him upright after the feed, or he might not. It isn't necessary to spend hours rubbing his back until he does so. It can be frustrating for you and uncomfortable for him – in fact he is liable to swallow air during this process rather than during the feed so will eventually burp anyway. If he doesn't settle when you put him back in his cot after the feed pick him up and see if he brings up any wind then, if not, put him back on the breast. Babies like to suck even if they aren't hungry any more and if you are tired you can always lay the baby down on the bed beside you as shown on page 44 and doze until he is asleep.

When your milk comes in

Mature milk starts to come in between thirty-six and forty-eight hours of delivery. You will probably notice the change from colostrum as your milk gradually becomes whiter and more watery. Many inexperienced mothers worry at this point since the milk does not seem to be as creamy as before and they think that it must therefore be less nutritious. This is a common misconception: mature breast milk is much thinner than colostrum, cow's milk or infant formula (although this is similar if made up properly). It contains everything that a baby needs in exactly the right proportions (see p. 11) and also provides enough fluid to quench your baby's thirst, even in very hot weather.

If you have been putting the baby to the breast every three hours or so milk comes in more quickly and you are less likely to become engorged. However, babies often don't feed that frequently at first so with a first baby the milk may not come in until the third or fourth day, and very many women find that suddenly their breasts are swollen and tender and the ducts behind the areola are full. Their nipples will probably leak milk.

Luckily by this time your baby's appetite will also be increasing. Feeding at this point needs fortitude. You may feel that your baby is constantly at the breast as he asks to feed as often as twelve or even fifteen times in twenty-four hours. Although this can be tiring, it is a temporary situation, lasting at most a week, during which time your baby will be emptying your full breasts and making them more comfortable, and helping to establish a balance between supply and demand.

If this is your first baby, during this time you need the support of the midwives, your partner and other more experienced breast feeding mothers who have gone through it before. It is not helpful if people say things like 'Feeding again?' or 'That baby obviously isn't getting enough if you have to feed that often.' Try not to take any notice of ignorant and unthinking remarks like these; they are likely to undermine your confidence and make you think there is something wrong with you or the baby when in fact you are both doing exactly the right thing. Your baby's appetite has increased after the initial quiet days after the birth; his weight will have dropped and he is busy replenishing stocks. You meanwhile are supplying them in abundance; if you don't let him feed when he wants to then that is when problems associated with engorgement set in (see p. 54).

When your breasts are very full you may need to express a little milk to enable your baby to grasp the areola as the milk collecting in the ducts behind it may make it rather enlarged. In addition your baby may splutter or choke a little on the unaccustomed first rush of milk. Supporting your breast from underneath with one hand, stroke downwards towards the nipple with the other, then hold your breast between forefinger and middle finger above the areola and squeeze downwards towards the nipple. This should release some of the milk which you can wipe away with a tissue before presenting your nipple to your baby.

Very full breasts, and large breasts generally, are sometimes difficult for a baby to feed from at first. Normally a baby has no difficulty in breathing during breast feeding even when he is pressed up quite close to your breast because his nostrils face downwards. Large breasts might be a bit overwhelming and, until he has got used to positioning himself in the right way, may impede his breathing, causing him to panic. You can get round this by supporting your breast from underneath with a hand held against your rib cage which lifts and elongates your breast, and helps the nipple to stand out more so that your baby can get a better hold. Another solution for full or large breasts is to lie on your side with the baby beside you as shown on page 44.

If your breasts do become uncomfortably engorged, and they can feel very hard, lumpy and hot, you can relieve the discomfort and soften the breast before a feed by holding warm flannels against them, or better still, lying in a warm bath. Expect some milk to leak; this is a good thing since it relieves the pressure behind the areola and makes it easier for the baby to latch on to the nipple. If your baby hasn't emptied the breast after a feed express the excess milk by hand or with a pump (see p. 69), or apply ice packs which will cause the distended blood vessels to contract. Your breasts may feel very tender when you lie down so don't let them flop about but wear a supporting bra at all times. Place breast pads inside your bra to catch leaking milk – the conical shaped ones fit most comfortably – but change them and your bra frequently.

Comfortable positions for breast feeding

Varying the position in which you hold your baby to feed is helpful both in preventing back ache or stiff shoulders and for avoiding sore nipples, since the baby will latch on at a slightly different angle each time.

The most common position to feed your baby is illustrated below, but it is important always to make sure that you and the baby are well supported with pillows because this method can result in back ache if you have to slump forward to enable the baby to reach the nipple.

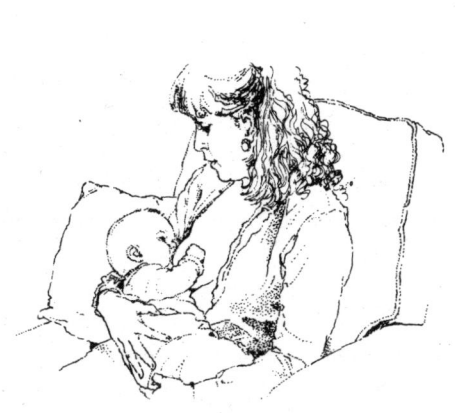

Positions for breast feeding

1   Cradle your baby in your arms using your hand to turn his body slightly towards yours. Support your back and elbow with pillows to avoid back ache. (Further positions overleaf.)

An alternative position if you are sitting up in bed and have aching shoulders is to place a pillow alongside you under your elbow and lay your baby on it tucked under your arm with his head in front. You can cradle his head with your hand or have both hands free to help him on to the nipple. This is helpful if you are a bit engorged as there is no danger

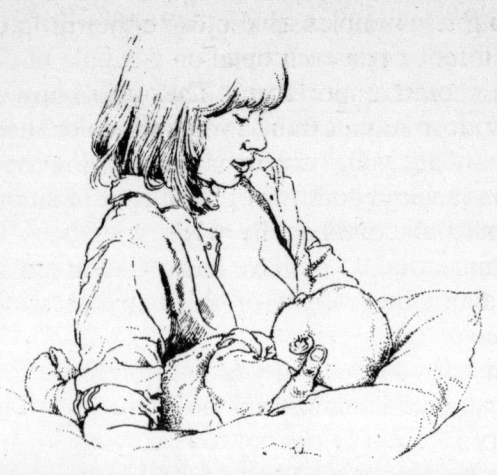

2 *Sit up with your baby tucked under your arm, again supported by pillows.*

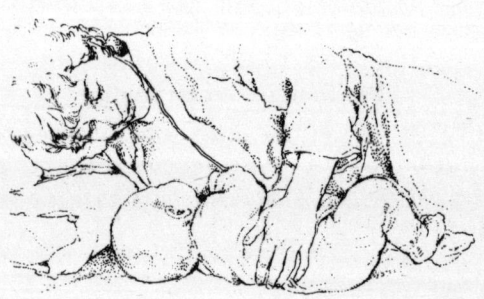

3 *Lie down with your baby lying beside you, he can then feed from the lower breast.*

of your baby's nostrils being covered.

Another and very restful way is to lay the baby on the bed beside you and lie on your side opposite him. He can then feed from the lower breast. You can either prop yourself up on your elbow or rest your head on a couple of pillows with your arm tucked under them. The upper arm can cradle your baby close to you. When you need to change sides you can sit up and lift your baby over, then lie down on the other side. This is a very good way of feeding at night because you can continue to doze happily while your baby feeds. It is also recommended if you have had a Caesarean section and want to avoid the weight of the baby pressing on your wound (see p. 65).

As your baby grows and you become more expert you'll find you can feed in almost any position. If you sit in a chair to feed, try to use a foot stool to raise your knees and take the baby's weight, again to avoid back ache. Another position that some mothers find comfortable is to sit cross-legged on the floor or on the bed, cradling the baby in the traditional way, with a cushion or pillow to raise the knee which is supporting your elbow under the baby's head.

FOUR

Problem solving

Although breast feeding should not be thought of in terms of problems, they undoubtedly do arise from time to time and the important thing to remember is that they *can* be solved. For first time mothers, the problems tend to arise in the first few days and weeks of feeding, but even the more experienced mother who has successfully fed one or two babies already may suddenly find that unexpected difficulties are presented with a subsequent baby.

Although obvious physical problems like blocked ducts or cracked nipples do occur and have to be dealt with, you may well have other worries which, although not as tangible, are none the less important, and need to be cleared up to enable you to feed your baby confidently. For instance you may wonder how you know if your baby is getting enough milk, or whether it agrees with him. It is hoped that by dealing with these common problems one by one, you will be reassured that you are not in any way different from other people and that whatever your particular difficulty, you can overcome it with patience and support. You may well find, too, that the solutions to different problems are very similar and there is lots of overlap in the explanations. This is because many are indeed simply variations on the same theme because the basic physiology of breast feeding is the same for all women.

Of course, it is easy to read about the solution to a problem – it is a different matter to put it into practice. This is where the help of a sympathetic midwife, health visitor or, especially, an experienced breast feeding mother can be invaluable. In the early weeks you will very likely be feeling physically tired, and the hormonal changes in your body will be turning you into an emotional roller-coaster. In this situation, difficulties with breast feeding can make you feel a total failure, so it is important to confide in someone whose advice you trust.

How fathers can help

Unhelpful or unsolicited 'advice' is one of the worst enemies of successful breast feeding, so if possible, you should try politely to ignore it. This is one area where your partner can be ready to fend off your next-door neighbour or your own mother when they start to bombard you with misleading statements. You may even find that you're putting a brave face on it to the midwives on the ward because they're so busy and you don't want to bother them with your trivial problems, only to dissolve into tears when your partner comes to visit you.

Fathers need to be ready for this eventuality; after the euphoria of the first day or two it can be disconcerting to find that your wife or girlfriend seems so miserable when you come to see her. In fact it is not because she is not pleased to see you or is unhappy with your baby. On the contrary, it is because she is probably feeling lonely and vulnerable and desperately needs your support. This weepy period may well coincide with the arrival of her mature milk, so she's probably uncomfortable as well. You can do more to build up her confidence than anyone by putting your arm round her and actively encouraging her to feed the baby when you are there. Everyone will benefit because she feels more relaxed, she'll cheer up and if there are difficulties with feeding, you can go and get the midwife and everyone can talk it through together as a shared problem.

Getting advice

Some of the problems which are explained here may crop up in the first week or two; others may well appear later on, when you're back home. This can be more unnerving than when you are in hospital; your partner may be out at work and you find yourself grappling with a fractious baby all by yourself. This is when those contacts you made during pregnancy become vital (see p. 10).

Don't sit alone in the house miserably trying to latch your baby on to a painful nipple or trying to cope while he refuses to settle to the breast or back to bed afterwards. Get in touch with someone who can give you immediate support, either on the telephone, or better still who can come round and see you or to whose house you can go. It may be your health visitor, or the breast feeding counsellor from your local National Childbirth Trust or La Leche League group, or the person from one of these groups who has agreed to act as your postnatal support. Or better still, it could be someone you know well, a relation or close friend, who is also a breast feeding mother or has been in the recent past. She will know exactly what you are going through, both physically and emotionally and will help with practical advice and a sympathetic ear. It is amazing what a relief it can be just to talk to someone you know really well who has been through it all before and won't think you are silly or exaggerating.

Enough milk

The inexperienced mother often worries to start off with whether she has enough milk for her baby. Because you can't see the milk coming through as you can from a bottle and you may not at first feel the characteristic tingling of the let-down reflex, you may even wonder whether any milk is coming out at all. Alternatively, you may have experienced the sensation of fullness, engorgement even, which lets you know that milk production has started, but then after a few weeks your breasts settle down and don't feel hard any more, so you may worry that they have suddenly stopped producing milk. On top of all this, your baby will lose weight in the first week – and the greater your baby's birth weight the more that weight loss is likely to be.

To reassure yourself that your breasts are producing milk, express a little from your nipple before you start the feed. If your baby latches on and suckles strongly there will be milk coming into his mouth – he would soon let you know if there wasn't (see below). Let him take his time, but when you feel he's had enough or it is time to change over, just pause and try expressing a little more milk from the breast he has just fed from. You will find that milk will still be produced from that breast. Remember that milk is produced all the time, and will be let down several times during a feed.

The time when the fullness caused by the start of milk production subsides should be accompanied by a huge sigh of relief rather than being an added source of worry. It means that your breasts are beginning to balance the amount of milk produced with the needs of your baby and is a good sign that breast feeding is established. It doesn't mean that your breasts have stopped producing milk as the test given above will prove. As has already been said, large breasts do not make more milk (see p. 26) and the enlargement due to pregnancy, and when milk production starts after the birth is temporary. In fact you may find that your breasts return quite quickly to their pre-pregnant size, and some women find that by the time their breast fed babies are about three months old, the mothers' breasts are actually smaller than before pregnancy.

Weight loss and gain

Whichever feeding method is used, all babies lose weight in the days after birth. It is nothing to worry about because they have reserves of fat to use up during this time (see p. 22). The progression from colostrum to a mixture of colostrum and milk and on to milk on its own is natural, and although you may see the baby in the next bed having milk from a bottle right from the start she is not going to do any better than your breast fed baby who follows this natural progression, even if she starts to regain her birth weight sooner.

It is true that the bottle feeding parent can see exactly how much his or her baby has taken, but this carries its own burden of worry. What if the baby doesn't drink it all? What if she drinks it all and doesn't seem satisfied? The temptation may be to encourage the baby always to finish the whole bottle, which could lead to an overweight baby, or maybe the mother will be faced with having to make up another feed (see p. 107). A breast fed baby takes as much as he wants and you know you can give him more without having to do anything special except put him back to the breast.

Your baby's appetite increases at the time the milk comes in and feeding becomes very frequent for a few days; this will almost certainly be accompanied by weight gain. Some years ago, babies used to be weighed daily in the hospital ward which was an added pressure for mothers. All babies are different, they all lose and put on weight at different rates and if one baby was losing more or gaining more than another it could result in unnecessary anxiety. Weight gain is now seen as only one of a number of factors indicating that a baby is thriving and developing normally and test weighing is only used when there is a specific reason which should be fully explained to you by the midwife or paediatrician.

You will probably find that your baby is weighed at birth, and then again at about five days old or when you are discharged from hospital. He will probably be weighed again by the community midwife looking after you at home at ten days old which is when she hands you over to the care of the health visitor. Babies have usually started to gain weight again between the sixth and tenth day after the birth, and while some return to their birth weights very quickly, others don't do so for two or three weeks, which is just a variation of normal. If you keep on feeding your baby when he is hungry and don't 'clock watch' while he is feeding you will be able to see and feel his weight gain. A visit to the clinic scales can be used simply as a useful corroboration of your own observations. Nowadays, overall developmental checks, plus general well-being and alertness are much better indicators of your baby's normal growth than just measurement of weight.

Just occasionally there may actually be insufficient milk so that your baby is frustrated and hungry. However, this is almost always a result of problems with the let-down reflex, not with the production of milk in your breasts as such. Problems with let-down are almost always to do with tension and worry, and can be as much the result of physical problems such as sore nipples or engorgement as of the sort of worries discussed above, so it is probably best to deal with the physical problems first.

Sore nipples

There may be initial tenderness when your baby first starts to breast feed while your nipples are still getting used to the strong suction. This is usually only in the first few seconds – once the milk starts to flow through there is no discomfort. If you had classes to prepare for labour, you can use the same techniques to breathe through those first few sucks, and this can also help if you experience after pains in the first couple of days following the birth.

If one of your nipples becomes really sore, so that it continues to hurt throughout the feed, your baby is probably not latched on properly and is chewing the nipple rather than gripping the areola with his gums. Check the position of his tongue, which should lie under the nipple, as well as that of his gums round the areola. If you aren't sure ask the midwife or another experienced breast feeding mother to check for you.

Check your baby's position in your arms too; he is much more likely to latch on properly if his whole body is turned towards your own rather than just his head (see p. 43). Vary the position you feed him as well, so that the main pressure of his gums isn't always on the same part of the areola.

If you are engorged and the nipple isn't protruding well because your areola is swollen with milk, express a little to start off with and support your breast underneath as described before (see p. 42) so that it is easier for your baby to latch on properly.

Try to avoid analgesic sprays or creams. These are off-putting to the baby and won't encourage him to latch on properly, so may exacerbate the problem. So long as a crack doesn't develop in the skin the soreness will subside when the baby is feeding properly.

Cracked nipples

If the soreness persists and is quite sharp and localized, you may have a tiny crack in the skin of the nipple. This may be invisible to the eye although the nipple may look rather red and angry, and there may even be a drop or two of blood. This can be very painful and really off-putting for the mother who is a bit tentative about breast feeding anyway. However, there should be no reason to stop breast feeding if you do develop a cracked nipple.

Cracks heal very quickly, within a day if dealt with promptly. Skin heals best if it is dry and open to the air, so stop wearing a bra as much as possible, or open the flaps of a nursing bra, and don't wear breast pads which keep the skin damp. Change your bra and clothes frequently if you are inclined to leak milk (see p. 54). If you've got the opportunity, expose your breasts to warm sunshine but be very careful not to become sunburnt. Don't however use a sun screen on your breasts. Wear underclothes or nighties made of cotton or other natural fibres rather than man-made fibres which tend to make you sweat.

When feeding take great care to make sure the baby is latched on properly. Persuade him to open his mouth wide to take the whole nipple in by making it protrude as far as possible (see p. 37) and use your breathing technique to get you over the first few sucks. Distract yourself with the radio or television, a cup of tea or good conversation.

A compress of ice cubes applied to the nipples inside a dry tissue really helps to ease nipple pain; apply it immediately before a feed. At the end of the feed don't drag your nipple out of the baby's mouth as this will simply open the crack and delay healing. Always release the suction with your finger so that he opens his mouth fully and you can withdraw your nipple in one go.

Don't use soap to wash your nipples, just clean them with plain water in your hands, rather than a face cloth or sponge which may introduce bacteria and set up an infection (see below). Once again, don't use antiseptic sprays or creams. Some may contain substances harmful to the baby and they mask the natural smell of the milk which encourages the baby to suckle. Anything which is likely to dry the skin will only encourage further cracking anyway, and will inhibit the natural lubricating action of the Montgomery's tubercles (see p. 27). However, there is no harm in taking a suitable pain-killer about half an hour before a feed if you think it may help. Ask your doctor's advice for a safe brand which will not harm the baby in the minute traces which inevitably enter the milk.

If it really is very painful to feed you could use a nipple shield for a few feeds although some babies find them a bit difficult to grip on. It is a good idea to express some milk into the shield first so he can taste it immediately he starts to suckle. It probably wouldn't do any harm to feed from the unaffected breast only for a couple of feeds, expressing as much milk as you can with a hand pump from the other.

Leaking

Leaking milk from the nipples is something that most breast feeding mothers have to contend with during the first few weeks and even later. Although it is inconvenient because it can stain your clothes it is in a way an encouraging sign because it means that you are making plenty of milk and that your let-down reflex is working.

You'll probably find that you leak in the first few days after the milk comes in because you are actually producing more milk than your tiny baby needs. You can collect this extra milk and freeze it for later use or donate it to the hospital milk bank. It will usually be the more dilute foremilk so while it is fine for quenching thirst, if you intend to collect a whole feed you should express properly with a pump to get the benefit of the calorie-rich hind milk, or your baby will not be fully satisfied (see p. 70).

Later on when your milk production balances with your baby's needs, leaking usually only occurs when you would normally be giving a feed but perhaps you are late back or you can't feed immediately because you are driving home from a visit. You may even find that your breasts leak just by thinking about your baby. Breast pads soak up the leaking milk efficiently, make it a habit to put one into your bra when you put it on and keep spares with you at all times. Don't leave a soaked breast pad in place for a long period as the damp makes your skin more liable to soreness and cracking. If you do have a crack, it could become infected with stale milk (see above).

Blocked ducts

Blocked ducts are caused by incomplete emptying of the ducts during feeds and occur most often, though not exclusively, during the first few weeks when your milk supply may still not have achieved equilibrium with your baby's needs. It could equally well happen when your baby is a lot older and changes his feeding routine, perhaps sleeping through the night and cutting out one or even two regular feeds quite suddenly, so that your breasts continue to produce milk but he is not emptying them when you expect him to.

Blocked ducts can also happen if your baby isn't correctly positioned on the breast so is not obtaining milk properly. You also run the risk of incomplete emptying of ducts if your baby is given complementary or partial bottle feeds at this stage so that he is not so eager to suck vigorously at the breast. Since this latter case is more likely if you are having trouble positioning your baby properly and he is still hungry and frustrated it could become a vicious circle of cause and effect. You may also block a duct by wearing a bra which is too tight, preventing the milk from flowing down the ducts where the pressure is greatest.

If a localized area of your breast becomes firm and tender, you should suspect a blocked duct. The swelling occurs when more milk is let down and pools behind the blockage. There is no need to stop feeding when this happens, on the contrary, it is really important to feed as frequently as possible from the affected breast to clear the blockage as soon as possible. Apply a hot flannel to the area to soften the tissue and gently massage it with the tips of your fingers in a downward direction. It is a good idea to put your baby to the affected breast first when he is hungry and will suck most vigorously. This will help to clear the blockage.

Mastitis

Mastitis is the name given to a bacterial infection in the breast. Some people mistake a blocked duct for mastitis, but although a blocked duct may eventually lead to infection if it isn't cleared, prompt attention as described on page 55 usually clears it before infection is allowed to set in. Mastitis may also be caused by bacteria entering the breast tissue through a cracked duct.

Mastitis should be suspected if you have a tender section of the breast which is also red and probably quite hot to the touch. The tenderness may extend up into your armpit, especially if the affected area is in the upper part of your breast. Your temperature will probably be raised and you may feel shivery, with swollen glands in the neck and a headache, symptoms similar to flu. If this is the case you should see the doctor as soon as possible so that you can be prescribed a suitable antibiotic.

You need to get plenty of rest, just as you would if you had flu, don't stop breast feeding because you have mastitis. The antibiotics won't harm your baby and continued milk flow is important as it maintains the blood flow to the breast which helps fight the infection. It is also important in that it avoids the development of a much worse condition, a breast abscess.

Breast abscess

This is quite rare but also quite serious. Just as some people mistake a blocked duct for mastitis, so a few others may mistake mastitis for an abscess and therefore stop breast feeding, so encouraging the very condition they ought to avoid. The symptoms of an abscess are similar but more acute than mastitis, and may be accompanied by pus leaking from the nipple. You will be treated with powerful anti-biotics and if the abscess is very bad it may mean admission into hospital to have it surgically drained.

An abscess is the only breast condition which means you have to stop feeding from the infected breast. However, milk flow has to be maintained as it helps to clear the infection more quickly, so you are well advised to express as much milk as possible from the affected breast, and then throw it away. You can continue to feed your baby from the other breast. Your doctor, health visitor or the hospital may well arrange for you to borrow or hire an electric breast pump until the abscess has healed (see p. 70).

You may worry that you won't have enough milk to feed your baby from one breast, but your body adjusts very quickly and although you may have to feed more frequently for a while you will provide enough milk for his needs. The real problem with a breast abscess is that it almost certainly has occurred because earlier problems have gone unresolved for too long. It also makes you feel quite ill, which in turn makes breast feeding less appealing, so it not surprisingly often results in the abandoning of breast feeding during the period of treatment. Fortunately, the condition is quite rare nowadays as mothers are becoming better supported. The best thing is to avoid the eventuality altogether by seeking help with any breast feeding problems you encounter as soon as they arise.

Problems with let-down

As has already been mentioned, many early breast feeding problems arise from or result in problems with the let-down reflex. The milk is there, it is being produced, but something is preventing it from being squeezed down the ducts towards the nipple. This may seem odd since it is a reflex, that is to say something that should happen automatically without you having to think about it (see p. 29). Unfortunately, like many functions controlled by the pituitary hormones it can also be affected by how you feel – your mood and emotions.

You or your midwife or doctor may suspect failure of let-down if your baby feeds for a while but still seems fretful and dissatisfied after the feed, and is perhaps not starting to regain his birthweight as soon as he should (see p. 49). The doctor will have ruled out any other underlying causes in the baby himself, such as an infection, before coming to this conclusion.

You may also notice that your baby's nappy is frequently not wet or only damp which shows he is not getting very much fluid. Although he may be getting some of the fore milk which builds up in the ducts immediately behind the areola, he is not getting the calorie-rich hind milk which is let-down during the feed and which relieves hunger rather than thirst.

It can be very discouraging for a mother to feel that she is not satisfying her baby, especially if she had already been worrying whether she would have enough milk in the first place. This is a self-fulfilling prophecy. If a mother worries that she won't have enough milk, the chances are that this worry may affect her let-down reflex, resulting in the very thing that she had been anxious about. It could also make her feel a failure into the bargain.

If you are tense about breast feeding the let-down reflex can be inhibited. This could be for one of the physical reasons discussed above – perhaps you have a sore or cracked nipple and you begin to dread the moment the baby latches on. You may have had problems with mastitis and have to take antibiotics and are worried about whether they are bad for your baby. Since both of these problems have probably occurred in the first place because your baby is not sucking properly with his gums over the areola (see p. 37), it is important to go back to basics and check this. Once he is sucking properly you will automatically feel more confident about breast feeding and let-down will occur.

Other sources of tension and stress can affect let-down as well. Perhaps you are worried about the family at home; maybe your birth was hard or tiring or you had to have a Caesarean and have the added burden of recovering from a major operation. Possibly you are a little embarrassed by breast feeding in front of other people, or maybe you don't really like the idea of breast feeding at all (see p. 16).

If you think any of these or similar psychological pressures apply to you, don't be afraid to talk it over with a midwife, relative or friend. Think about ways of removing the stress which is affecting you. If there are real problems at home which you can't resolve with your partner, or if you are a single parent, talk to the hospital social worker. Keep your baby with you all the time and put him to the breast whenever you feel like it. If you're shy about breast feeding at first, pull the curtains round the bed.

There are practical things you can do as well like expressing milk by hand and putting the baby to the breast as soon as milk comes through the nipple, or applying warm face cloths or lying a warm bath immediately before a feed to encourage the milk to flow. This has the added advantage of helping you to relax which is worth trying consciously to do when you put the baby to the breast; change your position and do it lying down (see p. 44) so there is no pressure or tension in your body. It may seem silly but it really does help literally to 'think' the milk down – imagine it flowing into your baby's mouth. You don't have to tell anyone you're adopting these strategies if you feel slightly embarrassed by them!

The sleepy baby

Some difficulties with breast feeding occur not because there is anything wrong with the way you are handling it but because of the baby himself. Although babies are born with the instinct to suck (see p. 32), if they are rather sleepy to start off with they may need a lot of encouragement to get started with breast feeding. A sleepy baby that doesn't wake for feeds is worrying even for the most confident breast feeding mother because he will not be doing what is necessary to stimulate her milk supply and may lose rather too

59

much weight himself, causing the doctor or midwives to feel that complementary bottle feeds are necessary for his well-being.

Don't let your baby sleep on for more than about three hours at first, however tempting it may be, especially when people congratulate you about how 'good' he is. Newborn babies need at least six and probably eight feeds in twenty-four hours to maintain their energy levels and replace body fat lost during the days while your milk is coming in. You also need to feed regularly to stimulate milk supply.

Sleepy babies may have been affected by the drugs used during your labour, such as pethidine. He will also be affected if you had to have a general anaesthetic perhaps for an emergency Caesarean delivery (see p. 64), and occasionally may be affected by an epidural anaesthetic. A long labour may tire a baby just as much as his mother, although he usually recovers after a few hours' sleep. Your baby will also be affected by drugs such as sleeping tablets which you are taking while you are breast feeding. It is usual for a premature baby or a baby with jaundice to be sleepy at first (see p. 73).

If your baby is sleepy and reluctant to feed, wake him up after two or three hours, and stimulate him by changing his nappy first. Don't wrap him up too tightly while you are feeding, and unless the weather is very cold, open the window. Hospitals can be very warm and soporific and this can affect babies just as much as adults! When you put him to the breast tickle his cheek with a finger to encourage him to open his mouth, and express a little milk onto his lips to encourage him (see p. 36). Hold him as upright as possible, supporting your arm with pillows. This is not a time to breast feed lying down. If he feeds for a bit and then falls asleep again, put him over your shoulder and carry him round the room for a bit, then try again.

Many babies fall asleep in the middle of a feed, especially

if they were very hungry and guzzled away for ten minutes. This is a great effort for them and it's not surprising that they want a rest, just as adults do between courses of a large meal. Your baby will soon let you know that he still wants some more when you move him, especially if you attempt to put him back in his cot. The sleepy baby, however, requires much more encouragement to get going again and you will need patience and perseverance. Once his appetite improves he'll be as demanding and wakeful as the next baby! However, if he seems very sleepy always get your doctor to check him in case he is unwell.

The resistant baby

Some mothers are disconcerted to find that their babies, who began breast feeding normally start to resist being put to the breast. The baby becomes stiff and arches his back, and will cry angrily, turning his head away from the breast, even though he is obviously hungry. This is a rather alarming phenomenon and sometimes makes mothers think that there is something wrong with their milk.

However, this is not the case. Some people think a baby becomes resistant because breathing was impeded by having his nose pressed up against the breast, but this is very unlikely as a baby's nostrils point downwards and so allow him to breathe even if he is being cradled very close. Whatever the cause, once again you need patience and perseverance to overcome this fortunately temporary behaviour pattern, using trial and error for the best method.

If your baby starts resisting the breast, first of all you need to calm him down. Lift him away from the breast and walk him round the room over your shoulder in an upright position. Perhaps your partner could do this to allow you to calm down too. Then you could try feeding the baby in a different position from the one which seems to upset him. Babies do seem to be calmed by stroking, so you could gently stroke his hair or his back while you guide him back on to the breast. If he has shown a preference for one side or the other, put him to the breast first on that side, even if it was first last time – there's no need to be rigid about these things when there's a problem to overcome. When you do move him over to the other breast keep his head in roughly the same position by tucking his body under your arm in the football position (see p. 44) rather than changing his whole alignment. Above all, try to relax and keep calm yourself; your mood will transmit itself to your baby and if you are tense he is more likely to be as well.

FIVE

Some special circumstances

There are some circumstances where breast feeding involves a bit more than simply presenting a breast to your baby and letting him nurse until he's had enough. If you have had a Caesarean birth, your baby was born prematurely, or develops jaundice, or perhaps you gave birth to twins, you can still feed your baby yourself but you may need extra help and advice at the start on the best way to achieve it for the well-being of both yourself and your baby or babies.

Although the above circumstances are less usual, there is no reason why breast feeding should not be successfully established for these babies. It may not seem so obviously easy if your baby is born with a congenital condition such as cleft lip or palate, but it is possible for highly motivated parents who want to give their baby the best possible start in life. Even babies who are found to be mentally handicapped, which can affect their basic sucking reflex, are breast fed by devoted mothers. With determination and a lot of support, there are almost no circumstances which prevent you feeding your baby with breast milk.

After a Caesarean
A Caesarean section involves major abdominal surgery which means that you will be far less mobile at first than

mothers who have had a vaginal delivery, even if they required assistance with forceps. If your operation was done under epidural anaesthesia, which means that you are not unconscious during surgery, you will feel better in yourself as it is less of a trauma than a general anaesthetic.

Either way, you will need lots of help, especially in the first forty-eight hours, both for your own needs and those of the baby. Some hospitals allow your partner, a close relative such as your mother or a friend to stay for the first couple of days to help you. Just turning over in bed has to be done with great care to avoid straining the incision, but a physiotherapist will show you safe ways to move around and will help you get mobilized as soon as possible. You'll also be given analgesics to ease the pain of the wound.

All this has a bearing on breast feeding. There is no reason why you should not breast feed your baby after a Caesarean. In fact, being able to feed your own baby can be a great morale booster if you feel disappointed that you weren't able to have a normal delivery. This is quite understandable, especially if the Caesarean is performed as a result of a last minute emergency.

If you had an epidural anaesthetic, and your baby is healthy after the birth, ask if you can put him to the breast for a minute or two in the recovery room. If you are lying on your side the midwife can bring the baby to you and you can let him latch on in the way described on page 44. However, if you had a general anaesthetic, or the Caesarean was performed as an emergency measure because there was concern over your baby's condition, perhaps after a long labour, neither you nor your baby are going to be able to start breast feeding for a few hours. You will feel drowsy for some time as you recover from the anaesthetic and your baby, who may also be sleepy from the effects of the anaesthetic, will probably be sent to the special care baby unit for a while for observation.

It is difficult not to worry under these circumstances, but even if your baby is given a bottle of milk – or more likely, glucose and water – during this time of recovery, it is not going to prevent you from breast feeding. Once both the baby and placenta have been delivered, the same hormonal activity takes place in your body no matter what method of delivery is undertaken, and although full lactation may be delayed for a day or two, you can still feed your baby.

While you are recovering from a Caesarean you need a great deal of rest and should drink lots of fluids. Once you and the baby are reunited you can concentrate on feeding, and let someone else do the chores such as changing nappies, clothes and bedding. This is why it's a good idea to have someone with you all the time because even lifting your baby at this stage can put undue strain on your wound if done without care. Feeding your baby lying down is both restful and comfortable since it doesn't put any weight on your wound at all, although turning over to feed from the other side can be difficult. Follow the instructions of your physiotherapist for turning over and sitting up. You should always take the weight on to your hands so that you do not contract the weakened stomach muscles and jeopardise healing. For this reason it is a good idea to offer one side only for a whole feed and be ready to lie on the other side for the whole of the next feed.

You may also find it comfortable to be sitting upright sometimes, well supported by pillows and with at least one light-weight pillow over your wound so that the baby does not press against it. Using the football position (p. 44) is another way of remaining upright but with no pressure on the wound. Don't worry about taking the pain-killers that you are offered. They won't harm your baby and they will make you more comfortable and therefore better disposed to feed your baby and do what is necessary to speed your own recovery.

Although you should probably stay in hospital for seven to ten days after a Caesarean, in practice pressure on beds means that you will probably go home after five days if you are making good progress, your baby is healthy and the doctors know that you have plenty of support at home. You must continue to rest as much as possible – don't be afraid to take your baby into bed with you (see p. 83). It is always difficult to be as 'selfish' as you should be about your recovery if you have older children. Explain as best you can about your sore tummy so that your toddler doesn't try and jump on your lap like she used to do, and keep yourself well padded with pillows in case she forgets!

Breast feeding twins

Contrary to what people may tell you, there is no reason why you should not breast feed twin babies if you have them. The extra stimulus from the second baby means that your breasts produce enough milk for both of them. It may require a bit more planning than breast feeding just one baby, but provided that both you and they are healthy the logistical problems are easily overcome.

If you know that you are expecting twins it is a good idea to discuss feeding with your doctor or midwife at one of your antenatal check-ups, so that your wishes are clearly stated in your notes. There is no doubt that twin births are subject to more intervention than singletons, with the result that both you and the babies are likely to be tired or require some special attention after the birth. This may involve some time for at least one of them in the special care baby unit (see p. 75). However, if the hospital staff are aware that you want to breast feed your babies (and your partner might have to remind them), then they can help you start and avoid giving bottles in the first day or so.

Starting to breast feed twins is no different from single babies (see p. 34), it just takes longer because there are two

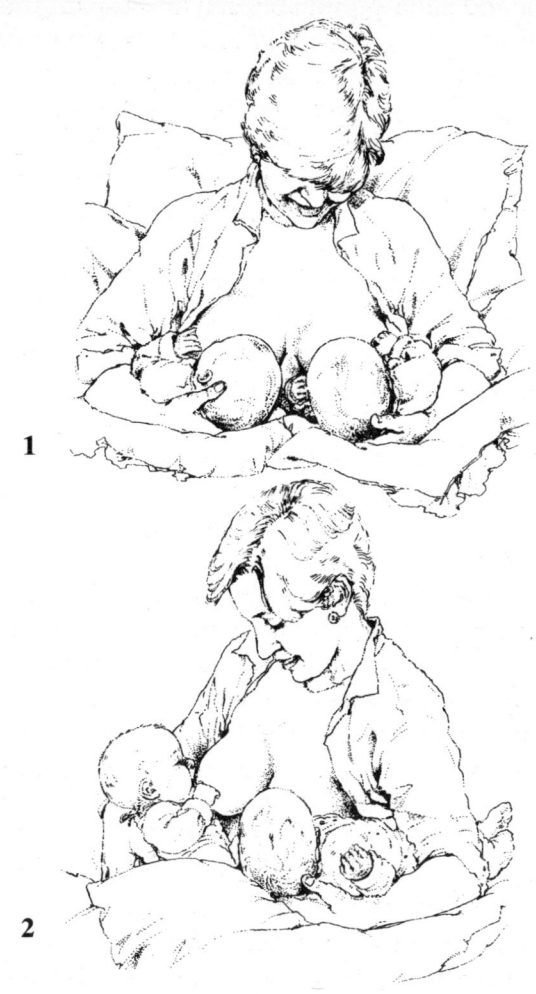

Positions for breast feeding twins

1 Tuck one baby under each arm with their heads supported on pillows.

2 Have one baby cradled in the conventional way and the other tucked under your other arm.

of them. Although it is probably a good idea to give the first few feeds separately so you can check that they are latching on properly, ultimately separate feeding is very time-consuming. Luckily you have two breasts so you can feed them simultaneously. The midwives will give you lots of help in the first few days and it is important that you get as much rest as possible. Breast feeding uses up 600 to 800 extra calories a day, breast feeding twins uses even more, so you should eat when you feel hungry and drink lots of fluids (see p. 84).

Positioning your babies when feeding simultaneously means propping yourself up with lots of cushions all around. You can either cradle one in each arm resting them on pillows across your lap and under your elbows, or have them both tucked under your arms in the 'football position' (see p. 44). Sometimes you could have one lying across and one tucked under your arm to vary the position of the babies' mouths on your nipples. Don't always keep the same baby at the same nipple, change them over between feeds. Twin babies grow at different rates and may have different sucking rhythms, and one baby is sometimes a little stronger than the other so they need to have a chance to suckle from either side in order for your milk supply to be balanced.

Sometimes you may like to feed one baby at a time in order to give each one that special individual cuddle. This is easy to organize if one baby wakes before the other, although if it is always the same baby that tends to wake first then you should occasionally change over and make that one wait. Alternatively, once breast feeding has been established, it will not do any harm to breast feed one baby and let your partner or a friend or relative give the other baby a bottle (see p. 108). If you have lots of milk you might even be able to express some to be given by bottle but most mothers of twins find this difficult to achieve. Feeding takes up quite a lot of time in itself, without spending more time expressing milk as well.

If you find there comes a time when there isn't help available, particularly during the day, and you want to feed the babies one at a time, no harm will come from introducing a dummy to pacify the waiting baby, if he will take it. You often find that one twin has a more placid personality than the other although try to avoid the temptation to exploit this – placid babies need just as much attention as demanding ones!

However, mothers who have breast fed twins successfully have found that breast feeding simultaneously is least time-consuming and less tiring in the long run, particularly if you have any older children to think of. On the whole, caring for twins is not twice as much work as looking after one baby, but only half as much again.

Even so, the majority of mothers of twins probably cease to breast feed at every feed by about three months either because they are becoming tired and feel very restricted or because they find that they simply aren't able to produce enough milk for their babies' needs after this time. There is no need to feel guilty if you feel like this yourself. Breast feeding twins is a major commitment and any mother who manages to breast feed for three months or more should feel proud of the achievement. Even if you could only manage for a few weeks, you know that you have given your babies the best start in life (see p. 13).

Expressing milk

There may well be occasions when you want to express some milk to be fed to your baby in a bottle, perhaps by someone else. The possibility of feeding one of your twins this way has already been mentioned above, and the mother of a single baby may prefer to do this if she wants to go out for a period of longer than three or four hours and doesn't want her baby to be given formula milk (see p. 94). You may have a baby in special care who isn't able to feed from the breast yet but can be fed your breast milk through a tube (see p. 75). Perhaps you find yourself in a situation where you have to express milk for a while which is discarded, possibly because of breast infection (see p. 55) or because you are taking some medication which would be bad for the baby, but you want to be able to breast feed again when the problem is solved.

Expressing a little milk at the beginning of a feed to whet your baby's appetite or relieve the pressure of very full breasts has already been discussed (see p. 41). In fact it often doesn't require any extra effort since your breasts may very well leak milk due to the early action of the let-down reflex. Expressing a whole feed is more time-consuming, especially if you are doing it by hand. You would only want to express by hand if you want to relieve engorgement, perhaps, or you have cracked nipples; otherwise, it is preferable to use a pump.

If you are only going to be expressing for perhaps one feed, you can use a hand pump which can be bought quite cheaply at chemists shops or baby care stores. There are several brands, but they all work on the principle of vacuum suction. The most usual type involves placing the trumpet shaped cup over your nipple and holding it firmly in place with one hand to create a vacuum. You then slide the other end of the pump backwards and forwards like a piston. The pressure of the cup against the areola and the action of the piston together draw the milk from your nipple into the pump.

Some designs can have teats fixed to the top directly so that they can be used as feeding bottles; with others the milk has to be transferred to a bottle for feeding. In both cases the pump should be sterilized in the same way as a feeding bottle to prevent any bacteria from entering the expressed milk. If the milk is to be fed to your baby within the next

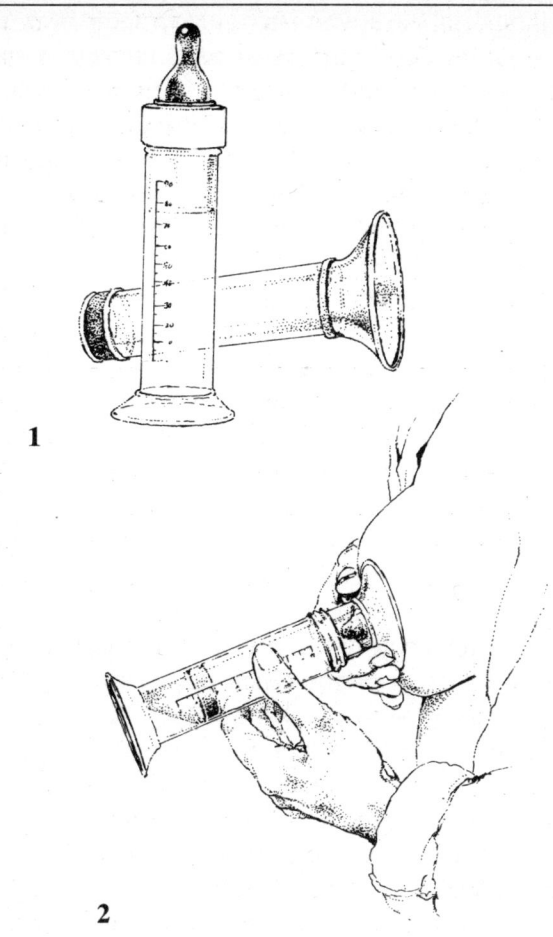

Expressing with a hand pump

*1   A typical hand breast pump which can be used as a bottle
for feeding.*
*2   Press the pump tightly against the breast to form a
vacuum. The lower half is then pumped backwards and
forwards to extract the milk.*

three or four hours, cover the container and keep it in the refrigerator until needed. If it is to be kept longer than that, the milk should be frozen immediately. If you are going to freeze expressed milk, it is a good idea to use the disposable plastic milk containers that come in a roll for use with a particular brand of bottle and teat (see p. 101). Place one of the bags inside the hand pump to catch the milk, then simply tie the end firmly with a freezer tie before freezing. Obviously, frozen milk must be completely thawed before it is given to your baby.

Expressing enough milk for a whole feed can take quite a time with a hand pump – a good fifteen to twenty minutes per side – so it needs perseverance. Having to express milk can interfere with the let-down reflex if it becomes a bore so if you find that you have to express milk for all feeds for several days, it is better to use an electric pump. This could well be the case if your baby has a poor sucking reflex or has to spend some time in the special care baby unit (see p. 74). Electric pumps can be hired or the hospital may be able to lend you one or allow you to use one in the unit.

An electric pump works on the same basic principle as the hand pump except that the suction is supplied by the machine. The milk collects in a sterilized beaker and is then transferred to another sterilized bottle or container for feeding or storage. Try to relax and sit comfortably while you are expressing milk and think about the good you are doing your baby by providing milk for him, especially if he is ill or premature. This will help the let-down reflex so that you are stimulating as much milk as possible.

You need to start expressing milk as soon as possible after the birth if your baby is born prematurely both to collect the protective colostrum for him and to stimulate lactation, just as you would if your baby were feeding directly from the breast. You will probably need to express milk at least four times a day for half an hour or more to maintain lactation, so once again you need to be highly motivated. If you can't keep it up for more than a few days, don't feel you are a failure. It is quite difficult to stimulate as much milk as your baby would if he was suckling direct and you may be disappointed by the apparently small amounts you manage to collect, especially at first. If you remember that you are doing it for your baby's well-being you can express milk successfully with an electric pump until he's strong enough to learn to breast feed himself (see p. 77).

The jaundiced baby

It is quite common for some newborn babies to become jaundiced in the first week of life. This doesn't mean that they have an infection such as hepatitis; although this might be possible it is extremely rare. It is much more likely to be physiological jaundice which is caused when the baby's immature liver cannot deal with the breakdown of red blood cells which is one of its main functions. When this happens the yellow colouring found in red blood cells, called bilirubin, accumulates in the bloodstream and tinges the baby's body with the characteristic yellowy-orange of jaundice.

This sort of jaundice often corrects itself within a few days without any special treatment, although more serious cases may be given phototherapy. The baby is laid naked in his cot under a special ultra-violet lamp with an eye mask to protect his eyes from possible damage. Phototherapy helps the baby's body to process the bilirubin more quickly. This treatment sometimes results in mild diarrhoea, but it passes when the treatment is completed.

Physiological jaundice affects the breast feeding mother because it can make a baby drowsy and slow to feed, while at the same time it is important that the baby's fluid intake is maintained. Some hospitals may suggest giving the baby bottles of water, but this isn't necessary if you are prepared to feed your baby at least every three hours. Your breast milk can provide all the necessary fluid but you will probably have to wake your baby up for feeds and he may require a lot of encouragement, probably falling asleep in the middle. It is worth persevering however as generally the condition clears after a few days and your baby will regain his appetite and normal alertness.

Nowadays, most phototherapy is carried out in the postnatal ward with a portable light suspended over your baby's cot next to your bed. This makes the frequent feeding easier as the baby is with you all the time.

Babies in special care

Although a full-term pregnancy is said to be forty weeks, in practice it can vary and even if your baby comes three weeks early, at thirty-seven weeks, so long as he seems healthy, has a well-developed sucking reflex and probably weighs more than about 4 lb 6 oz (2 kg) he won't be treated any differently from a full-term baby. He'll stay with you in the postnatal ward and breast feeding can proceed in the normal way.

However, if he comes significantly early, at thirty-six weeks or less, if the paediatrician considers him to be 'small for dates' or if he has any problems with breathing or feeding you may find he is taken to the special care baby unit or neonatal intensive care unit to be cared for by expert staff with specialist equipment.

Problems with metabolism

A very few babies have serious problems with their metabolism, their ability to digest and process milk for energy, growth and development. Every baby is now screened at about six days old for the most common of these conditions, called phenylketonuria (PKU). A blood test involving a tiny pin prick in the baby's heel can fortunately discover this condition and your baby will probably have to be given a special formula which doesn't contain a certain type of protein found in breast milk. This is disappointing for parents who had hoped to breast feed but it is reassuring to know that your baby can grow up normally – the consequences of this condition going undiagnosed could be disastrous.

Premature babies

Babies born before about thirty-six weeks are usually referred to as premature; one of the signs of prematurity is a poorly developed sucking reflex. Although babies do make sucking movements with their mouths, they are unable to suck a bottle or nipple to obtain milk until they are about thirty-three weeks' gestation, and even then may not be able to suck well enough to feed solely from the breast or bottle until they are the equivalent of thirty-five weeks or so, and in some cases as much as thirty-eight weeks. So if your baby is born early he will have to be fed through a tube inserted into his stomach through his nose, and if he is born at say thirty-two weeks of pregnancy, then you can expect this tube feeding to continue for at least three weeks. This doesn't mean you can't feed him yourself. In fact the best food for most premature babies is mother's milk, so you can contribute to his well-being by expressing your own milk which can then be fed to your tiny baby in the incubator.

All premature babies spend some time in the special care baby unit. Babies born early are very vulnerable to infection, to changes in temperature and sometimes have breathing problems because their lungs are immature. They must be kept very warm as they don't have the extra layer of insulating fat that the full-term baby is able to build up during the last weeks of pregnancy. They often need extra oxygen or even help with their breathing through a ventilator since a steady supply of oxygen is vital to their whole development, and especially their growing brain cells. The tiniest babies need constant surveillance and tests so will be wired up to high tech equipment and have tubes and electrodes attached to them so they can be permanently monitored by the expert staff.

A baby that has been born early has been deprived of the protective functions of the uterus and placenta which have to be provided instead by doctors, nurses and machines. The achievements of the neonatal intensive care units are extraordinary, as they are capable of looking after tiny babies weighing perhaps as little as $1^3/_4 - 2$ lb (800-900 g) who are born as early as twenty-four or twenty-five weeks. The whole situation can be very distressing for parents, especially as preterm births are often completely unexpected. Nowadays you will be encouraged to spend as much time as you can in the special care unit with your baby, helping the nurses care for him and above all being encouraged to provide your own milk to feed him with.

Tube feeding consists of running a fine sterile tube through your baby's nose directly into his stomach, which is attached to a small drip feed hanging above the incubator. Preterm babies have to be fed little and often so the more milk you can produce the better. As your baby begins to thrive you may be able to take him out of the incubator and hold him while the tube feed is being given. Gradually he will learn to suck, and may be given the feed in a bottle with a special teat.

However, if you want to breast feed the staff will probably advise you to persevere with the expressing and tube feeding until your baby is really ready to be put to the breast. This can be frustrating as it could be several weeks or even months before he reaches this stage and you can expect your milk supply to diminish since expressing milk is no substitute for a baby suckling and with the best will in the world it is difficult to keep it up. Don't worry; provided you can express a little regularly and you keep thinking about the good it is doing your baby, you will find that lactation soon returns to full strength once your baby is strong enough to feed solely from the breast.

Sometimes a baby may be born too early even to be able to absorb breast milk and may have to be fed with a special solution through a tube that leads straight into a vein. Even so you can express your own milk so that it can be frozen or given to the special care baby unit milk bank for other babies, and you can be ready to provide breast milk for your own baby when his stomach is mature enough to take it.

Some neonatal paediatricians prefer to feed certain premature babies with a special high calorie formula which enables babies to put on weight faster. If it is suggested that this would be better for your baby, and you are anxious about it, speak to the consultant in charge of your baby about the pros and cons. It may be that a mixed regime of the special preterm formula and your breast milk would be possible. Certainly breast milk contains the substances which can protect your preterm baby from dangerous infections and is particularly easy for the immature baby's stomach to digest, but if you are finding it difficult to express enough milk for his needs it may be better to allow the formula to be given to him while you continue to express. As long as it isn't being given to him in a bottle it won't interfere with successful breast feeding being established in the long run.

Getting your baby to take the breast once he does seem mature enough and ready to suck takes time, but if you have had the determination to express milk for several weeks it won't be difficult to summon up the necessary motivation to help your baby learn to suck. For the first few times he may only nuzzle the breast and in actual fact the feed is still given by nose, but if you express a little milk on to your nipple he will gradually learn that that is where it is coming from. He may only suck three or four times but you will know they are the real thing, and he will increase them at each feed as he grows stronger.

Some people suggest running the tube along your breast so that the end is by the nipple so that the baby learns to associate milk with your breast even though he can't suck vigorously. This may delay things however if the tube is then removed and the baby finds it very hard to obtain milk, so becoming frustrated and angry.

At this time of transition the more often you can feed your baby the better, and you may be invited to come and stay in the unit for a few days, especially if you live some distance from the hospital. However, it is a very happy time because it usually means that your baby is almost ready to come home.

Physically and mentally handicapped babies

The main physical handicap in a newborn baby which interferes with breast feeding is a cleft palate. This condition is obviously distressing for parents, but you will be reassured by the paediatricians at the hospital that it can be surgically corrected. However, this cannot be done until a baby is several months old, and in the meantime you may want to breast feed your baby.

The problem for a baby with a cleft palate is that it cannot maintain suction on the nipple along the roof of the mouth, and milk sometimes comes back down his nose causing him to splutter and sneeze. A special plate can be made to fit over the baby's palate to allow him to suck, or else a mother can be encouraged to express milk (see p. 69) and feed it to the baby on a spoon. This is time-consuming but babies become quite expert at it. A simple cleft lip doesn't usually interfere with sucking.

Certain types of mental handicap result in babies being unable or unwilling to suck, and this too, causes problems if you wish to breast feed. However, lots of mothers of handicapped babies are determined to breast feed, realizing that it is a way to come as close as possible to their vulnerable babies. In both these cases it is very useful to be in contact with the various self-help groups which can put you in touch with parents who have overcome similar problems (see Useful Addresses p. 125).

After a stillbirth

Today parents of stillborn babies are given a lot of support – you will both benefit from expert counselling to help you work through your grief. The onset of lactation is particularly hard to bear if your baby is stillborn or dies within the first week of the birth. Unfortunately, there is no way that your hormones can 'switch off' the process of lactation after the birth, even if your baby dies. Mothers who are suffering the bitter disappointment of the bereavement still have to go through the discomfort of milk coming in and probable engorgement with no baby to feed.

Your doctor may prescribe a drug to suppress lactation if that is what you want. Otherwise the best advice is to do nothing which will stimulate your milk supply once it comes in. An old-fashioned method which still has relevance is to bind your breasts tightly, although this is uncomfortable when they are tender and engorged. Wear a supportive bra as much as possible, with breast pads to catch leaking milk and hopefully lactation will subside within a few days.

SIX

Breast feeding and family life

Although this isn't a book about all aspects of baby care, breast feeding is so central to your baby's well-being that it can't help but influence the way you look after him. When you come home from the hospital, your baby is going to have an impact on everyone's life. If he's your first baby, you went into hospital as a couple and come back home as a family. If he's an addition to the family, his needs and his personality have to be accommodated with everyone else's. Breast feeding generally helps this transition as it is so flexible.

Looking after yourself

In the early days at home after the birth you do need to think about your own health and well-being. Looking after a tiny baby is tiring, whether you are breast or bottle feeding. Even if you've had four or five days in hospital, you may still be feeling tired or sore after the birth, and your baby may well be feeding every two or three hours. Even if he is managing four hours between some feeds, it still means night times broken by one or more feeds. Night feeds often continue for several months; few babies sleep right through the night before they are about six months old and many continue to wake well into toddlerhood.

It is a great help if your partner can take some time off work when you come home from hospital, or if you can enlist the help of active grandparents, or perhaps your sister or a close friend. If you don't have to worry about shopping, cooking and cleaning at least for a week or two it gives you a chance to regain your strength and get used to looking after your baby at home and build your self-confidence. As your baby is likely to change his routine when you get home and you yourself are having to cope without the midwives to fall back on when you're not sure of yourself, it does make things easier if you have help at hand during this rather vulnerable period.

You will of course be visited by the community midwife at home until your baby is at least ten days old, after which she will hand over your care to the local health visitor and your family doctor. The health visitor's job is to give advice and moral support. She is a nurse who has had extra training in the care and development of young babies and she will be based either in your doctor's surgery or at the local well baby clinic, where you can visit her or telephone her for advice on breast feeding or anything else that worries you or you are not sure about.

If you have been in touch with your local National Childbirth Trust, La Leche League or Association of Breastfeeding Mothers group, you will probably be contacted by another mother from the group who will offer postnatal support. This can be very valuable because these mothers will have experienced just the same joys and agonies that you may be experiencing with your baby. These organizations also train special breast feeding counsellors and you can ask to speak to your local counsellor if you are having specific problems with breast feeding. Even if you weren't involved in the groups before the birth, if you do need help you can always contact them afterwards and enlist their help.

Getting enough rest

You will find that everyone involved in caring for new mothers and babies is always urging you to rest. This can seem to be a tall order when your partner has had to return to work, your mother lives 200 miles away and you've got a home to run and an apparently insatiable baby to feed. This is when you really need to sit down with your partner and decide on the priorities. If you rush around trying to do everything just as you did before the birth you will soon find that your milk supply is being adversely affected and your baby will become fractious and hungry, asking to be fed even more frequently and therefore giving you even less time to yourself.

■ First of all, having a spotlessly tidy home is not important when your baby is small. You'll probably find you're spending most time in the kitchen, bathroom and bedroom, and as long as you're reasonably well-organized to start with and that you pay some attention to hygiene when washing and changing your baby, the rest of your home can get dusty. No one but you is probably in the least bit bothered by it anyway.

■ Babies do generate a lot of washing; a breast fed baby's stools are quite soft and watery and often stain clothes as well as nappies. Make sure you have plenty of spare stretch suits and vests, blankets and sheets so that you can have a big wash once or twice a week instead of every day. Don't bother going to the expense of buying extra clothes new – second hand clothes are just as good and you'll probably find them on offer cheaply at your local clinic, or there's bound to be a mother happy to hand down first-size clothes at least on a long loan.

■ While you've got help in the home, go back to bed and sleep whenever you feel like it and hand over the chores to your partner or helper. When you're on your own, go and lie down whenever you've got the opportunity. It won't be long before you discover that your baby has a particular time of day that he sleeps for slightly longer than at other times. If it's after the early morning feed, you can go back to bed too. If it's in the afternoon, you can lie down then as well.

■ Keep your baby's cot in the bedroom with you for the first few weeks. When he wakes at night you can lift him into bed with you and feed him lying down (see p. 44). It doesn't matter if you both fall asleep, you won't squash him. It has been proved that, provided neither partner has had any drugs such as sleeping tablets or been drinking alcohol, adults always roll away from a baby sleeping in bed with them.

In fact there are people who advocate the idea of the family bed in which parents and all children sleep together until the children are old enough to choose to sleep in their own beds. While this may not be everyone's choice, it is certainly a sensible option to have your baby sleeping beside you, or at least as close to you as possible while you are breast feeding at night, since it causes the least disturbance to everyone involved.

■ It's sensible to let your baby sleep in a carry cot or Moses basket so he can be where you are. This means you can pick him up to nurse as soon as he is ready. If your home is on more than one level, keep a set of baby changing equipment downstairs so that you don't always have to run up and down when he needs changing or he wakes for a feed. You will probably think of various other ways of saving yourself time and effort around the house.

■ Although visitors are a lifeline when you're at home with a small baby, too many can actually be a burden, so don't feel you have to 'entertain' them when people come to see you and the baby in the early weeks. Most people will be only too happy to make a cup of tea or coffee if asked politely.

Your diet

In general there is no need to eat or drink any more than usual while you are breast feeding, although equally it is not the time to start a slimming diet. This is unnecessary as well as bad for you. During the latter weeks of pregnancy you will have laid down extra fat to provide the calories required for lactation and these will be used up in the first weeks. This is a very efficient way of getting your figure back after the birth; some women find that breast feeding combined with the activity of motherhood means they end up feeling fitter and weighing less than they did before they were pregnant.

However, while there's no need to eat more, you should eat when you feel hungry and what you eat should be nutritious. You should aim for a good balance of meat and fish, dairy produce and eggs, fresh fruit and vegetables and dietary fibre, such as wholemeal bread, pulses and brown rice. If you are a vegetarian, you need to be especially careful to provide enough protein in your diet and you might be advised to take vitamin B_{12} supplements, particularly if you are a vegan.

You may also find that you feel less tired if you eat little and often, rather than relying on one large meal in the evening. Parents of young babies are often advised to rely on 'convenience foods', but this doesn't mean you have to stock up on expensive items from the chill counter or freezer section of the supermarket. Interesting sandwiches and rolls, fruit such as apples and bananas, nuts and salads, are all 'convenience' foods which require little preparation, and a filling Chinese take-away or even fish and chips are very nourishing. It might be an idea to avoid very spicy Indian food for a while, since what you eat or drink does affect your baby through your milk and occasionally you may find that certain foods result in runny stools or fretful behaviour the next day!

It is also unnecessary to drink large amounts. If you feel thirsty, have something to drink but don't force yourself. Drinking milk doesn't affect your own milk supply, so if you don't particularly like it, don't make a special effort to drink it. Make sure you are maintaining your calcium intake in others way, through cheese, yoghurt and green vegetables. Anyway, if your baby has been shown to have a cow's milk allergy (see p. 15), you may be advised to avoid cow's milk products until the baby is older.

Having said that, it is relaxing to sit down with a cup of tea or coffee, or a soft drink, beside you while you feed your baby. Feeding should be relaxing, and is a perfect excuse for putting your feet up. You benefit by resting your body, which helps lactation and let-down (see p. 29), and your baby benefits by being able to feed comfortably at his own speed.

Fathers and breast feeding

Behind every successful breast feeding mother there is usually an extremely supportive father. It makes a tremendous difference to a new mother if her partner is encouraging her efforts and sympathizing when things are a bit difficult. Some new fathers occasionally feel a bit redundant when their partners are breast feeding, but in fact your role is a very positive one. Particularly at first, when she is feeling a bit vulnerable, your partner will really appreciate the security you can give her just by being there and keeping her company while she is feeding.

Even if you didn't do much in the home before the birth, or you have to go out to work much of the week, try to take on more of the chores during the first few weeks and months while your baby is still tiny. Some men simply don't realize how time-consuming feeding can be until they experience it, but once you have appreciated this you can help your partner in so many ways – by going to the supermarket, taking on some of the cooking and tidying and above all keeping visitors at bay. Alternatively, you may feel that breast feeding keeps you apart from your baby, but you can contribute a lot more than you may think to your baby's care by taking over when he has finished feeding, by cuddling him, rocking him to sleep and by bathing and changing him.

You need to be extra tolerant of your partner's mood changes, too. If at the start she seems irritable or close to tears for no obvious reason, remember that both physically and emotionally she is going through momentous changes, and she's having to cope with these when she is also not getting enough sleep. This is not to say that you aren't too; in fact this is something which is too often overlooked. Fathers have broken nights and worry about their babies too, but it is worth both of you remembering that parenthood is a shared experience and that as always talking things through together – the achievements as well as the difficulties – helps to keep things in proportion.

Feeding and sleeping

Whether you feed by breast or bottle, there is a tendency for inexperienced parents to get the impression that babies simply feed and sleep. Although young babies do spend up to two-thirds of any twenty-four hour period asleep, it can seem a lot less than that because it doesn't happen at predictable times or when you yourself want to sleep. Right from birth babies have wakeful times when they may or may not cry.

Some babies sleep for three or four hours solidly in perhaps one or two periods during twenty-four hours, while the rest of the time they 'catnap' for half an hour or so, or may have quite long periods when they are fretful – crying for a while, perhaps sleeping when rocked then waking again. Other babies are placid and sleep regularly – these babies are often said to be 'good' while wakeful babies are some-times referred to as being 'naughty'. It's best to avoid these sort of terms when thinking about your baby. A small baby is incapable of being good or naughty in any real sense of the words – these are things which are learned at a much later stage when they begin to socialize.

Babies don't have any idea of the difference between night and day when they are small; a baby wakes at night for the same sorts of reasons he wakes in the day. You will soon be able to distinguish between different types of cry (see page 88). When your baby wakes at night for a feed, you can begin to show him that night times are different by not giving him any special attention beyond what is absolutely essential. Feed him in bed with you, change his nappy with the minimum of disturbance and put him back in his cot. If you put him in a double strength nappy and liner, or better still a terry towelling nappy, you can quite happily leave it on providing it hasn't leaked onto his clothes or bedding. Babies don't usually mind having a wet nappy so long as it isn't making them cold, although a soiled nappy should always be changed since it could result in a nappy rash.

When your baby wakes and cries, or won't settle after a feed, it may not be because he is hungry. You could try burping him, but in point of fact this is rarely the root of the problem, and if he has been crying for some time and then burps it is probably because he has swallowed air while cry-ing. Check whether he is wet and therefore cold, or has soiled his nappy, and that he is neither too warm nor too cold. Do this by feeling inside his clothes rather than by the temperature of his face or hands, but in any case a baby shouldn't sleep in a room temperature of less than about 60°F (15°C) and warmer when he is newborn. You can experiment with sleeping positions too; some babies prefer to lie on their stomachs, while others seem to be more com-fortable on their sides. Some babies also seem more secure if they are tightly wrapped in a blanket.

If after all these checks your baby still seems reluctant to settle, pick him up and give him a cuddle, and don't be afraid to put him back on the breast. He may simply want the comfort of sucking for its own sake, which gives babies a great deal of pleasure. After all many babies find their own thumbs to suck at a very early age, which can be a great relief to parents!

Of course, he may simply want to be awake and take notice of his surroundings. From about three weeks of age there is no reason why you should not put your baby into a bouncing chair near where you are so he can see and hear what you are doing. He'll soon let you know when he is really tired and may fall asleep in the bouncing chair anyway.

Feeding and crying

Feeding, sleeping and crying are very closely related. A baby will cry because he is hungry or thirsty, but he may also cry because he is uncomfortably wet, is too hot or cold, is unwell or simply because he is lonely or bored. He will also cry because he is tired.

While your baby is small it is sensible for him to sleep in the room with you (see above), but babies can be rather snuffly and disturbing even when they are asleep, so it may suit you better to have him nearby but not actually in the room if he is keeping you awake unnecessarily. There is no reason why you shouldn't put his carrycot just outside the door, so long as it isn't draughty, while you're still doing regular night feeds, or in another room close enough for you to easily hear his cries.

Parents, especially mothers, find they wake very easily when their babies cry, and can distinguish their baby's cry from another's within a few days of birth. You'll soon be able to tell whether your baby is crying from hunger or is in real distress. You can leave a hungry baby crying for a few minutes without any real problems, for instance while you change his nappy or make yourself a quick cup of coffee, but don't leave him bawling for ages simply because you think he can't possibly be hungry yet (see p. 38).

If your baby wakes frequently during the night, and won't settle to sleep for more than an hour or so at a time, you might be tempted to switch to bottle feeding in the hope that it will make him sleep for longer periods. While the occasional bottle given by your partner to allow you to rest isn't going to matter, it's a mistake to believe that bottle feeding is going to affect your baby's sleep pattern overnight. It is unlikely to make any difference because bottle fed babies are just as prone to wakefulness as breast fed ones and you will have given up the benefit and general convenience of breast feeding early for no reason.

There is no doubt that a constantly crying baby can be very trying and causes tension in a family. This is especially hard on the inexperienced breast feeding mother who could become anxious and depressed as nothing seems to settle her baby. This can have an adverse effect on the let-down reflex, setting up a vicious circle of cause and effect – the baby cries a lot, the mother becomes tense, the amount of milk the baby is getting reduces, and the baby cries more.

You can avoid this pattern by trying to keep in mind all the time that it is not your fault that your baby cries – it is just that some babies cry more than others. If your baby is pacified by being put to the breast, then do so. It will help him feel more secure and you can have the confidence of knowing that you are providing the best possible comfort for him.

If he seems to want to be carried all the time, use a baby sling so that he has the comfort of closeness and you have your hands free to get on with other things. Get out and about with the pram or buggy – movement often pacifies a fretful baby. Parents have been known to take their babies for long car rides at one o'clock in the morning simply to get them off to sleep! Above all share the burden; go and see a friend with a baby and compare notes or talk to your breast feeding counsellor or health visitor. If things are very difficult there is a support group which could help you (see Useful Addresses p. 125). Keep in the back of your mind that this is temporary – it may seem to be a cliché, but this really is 'only a phase he is going through'. If however you have reason to believe there is more to it, and that your baby might be unwell, don't hesitate to go to your family doctor. You shouldn't feel you are worrying unnecessarily; if there is nothing intrinsically wrong your doctor will be only too happy to put your mind at rest.

'Colic'

Some young babies develop a pattern of behaviour which involves long periods of crying, often in the afternoon and evening, during which they may scream and draw their legs up towards their bodies. Babies who do this are sometimes said to have colic, or be colicky, although this is a slightly misleading term. No single cause has been found for this very common situation, which often starts when a baby is three or four weeks old and then passes at about three months.

It is particularly difficult for parents to cope with when it happens at the end of the day, when you both are probably at your most tired, and if one parent has been at work all day, what you really want is each other's uninterrupted company for a while.

It is important to keep in mind that this is a temporary situation – babies do grow out of it. Apart from the advice given above, rocking, walking about with the baby over your shoulder, lying him across your knee and rubbing his back, are all strategies that have been found to give babies temporary relief. A little gripe water on a spoon may help although it is important never to exceed the correct dose. Find a competent baby-sitter and go out together in the evening. It is probably best to distract yourselves with a film or play rather booking a candlelit dinner during which the two of you fret constantly about whether your baby is all right.

If you feel depressed

Dealing with a young baby, especially the first time, is a big responsibility and sometimes it can make you feel lonely and depressed. If you were working before the baby was born, you may now feel isolated and restricted. Life may seem like a dreary round of feeding, changing, washing and broken nights. This is not a mood conducive to successful breast feeding – your emotions anyway have an effect on lactation (see p. 57) and mothers often give up breast feeding because they mistakenly believe that bottle feeding will give them more freedom. Making contact with other parents in the same situation who live nearby is very important, and even just going to the shops every day helps to avoid feeling house bound, so it's worth making the effort.

However, if you feel really depressed and unhappy talk to your health visitor or doctor. It is possible that there is a physical cause. You may, for instance, be anaemic and need to take iron supplements and look more carefully at the balance of your diet (see p. 84). Extreme tiredness can make you depressed. If you are getting very little sleep and are having to cope with older children as well, it might be an idea if you hand over the baby to your partner for a night or so, letting him give a bottle of expressed milk or formula just for one feed. If your breast feeding is well established this won't affect lactation. Alternatively you could go to bed as soon as he comes home from work, say at seven o'clock, and let him do everything else with the baby, just bringing the baby to you when he needs feeding. It's amazing what a lift you can get just from one decent night's sleep.

Real depression is something different – women do suffer from it after childbirth, although it may be weeks before it really manifests itself. This is more than the 'baby blues' which are the inevitable consequence of the hormonal changes, physical fatigue and domestic upheaval involved. Fathers are often the best people to note the serious signs. If your partner is very listless, loses her appetite and wants to sleep a lot, and seem to have little interest in life or her new baby, then she may need special treatment, and you should talk to your doctor without delay (see Useful Addresses p. 125).

Resuming love-making

Some couples are uncertain about resuming love-making when the mother is breast feeding. Under normal circumstances you are safe to resume sexual intercourse when you no longer have any vaginal discharge (lochia) after the birth. This will probably be within two or three weeks; check with your doctor if you are not sure. In any case if you are at all uncertain your doctor will be able to set your mind at rest at the postnatal check-up six weeks after the birth.

However, some couples find that love-making while the mother is breast feeding rather inhibiting. Your breasts during these early weeks may well be tender, which means that you may find it uncomfortable to have any weight put on them. In addition, you might find that they leak a little when stimulated, which can be a bit surprising and even off-putting if you're not expecting it.

However, breast feeding is not a reason for avoiding love-making. Find different and comfortable positions for intercourse, perhaps with the woman on top for a change or lying side by side, which don't put any pressure on the breasts. You need to take things easily and carefully to begin with anyway especially if you had stitches and you are worried that any activity might make you a bit sore.

Breast feeding and fertility

Breast feeding is a natural form of contraception; while you are breast feeding fully, the action of the hormone prolactin suppresses ovulation and you may well not have a period for six or eight months. However, it's not a good idea to rely on this as a completely safe method of contraception.

Your doctor or family planning clinic nurse can advise you on the best method of contraception while breast feeding. You could have a coil (IUCD) fitted at your postnatal check-up, use a barrier method (condoms or a diaphragm, which again needs to be fitted at your postnatal check), or take a progestogen-only pill (the 'minipill') which doesn't affect lactation.

If you do become pregnant again while you are still breast feeding, you might wonder whether you can continue to breast feed your older baby. Most women have ceased breast feeding by the time their babies are 12 months old, so the situation arises fairly infrequently, but for those mothers who do let their toddlers continue to nurse well beyond this age, it does seem to be possible (see p. 119). These children will only be suckling for comfort, not nourishment, so the natural suppression of lactation that occurs during pregnancy does not matter, and some mothers seem happy to continue to allow their toddlers to nurse even when they have a newborn baby at the breast as well.

The active mother

If you are a keen sportswoman, you may wonder when you first start lactating and your breasts are large and tender, whether you are ever going to be able to get back to your former active self. During the first few weeks any activity involving running or jumping may make your breasts feel uncomfortable.

Your breasts do settle down after a few months, losing their initial enlargement and becoming normally soft again. In any case, your doctor or physiotherapist at the hospital will probably advise you to resume exercise and sport very gradually after the birth, concentrating at first on getting your stomach and pelvic floor muscles back to normal strength after the stretching of birth. The hormones of pregnancy which allow your muscles and ligaments to soften and stretch continue to have an impact on your body up to five months after the birth so you have to be careful not to put undue strain on yourself, particularly on your back.

Get back into trim by swimming, cycling and the programme of postnatal exercises suggested by your physiotherapist. Invest in a couple of proper sports bras to give you extra support until your breasts are less tender.

Getting out and about

In many ways, breast feeding gives mothers more freedom to get out and about than bottle feeding. There is nothing extra to carry about with you and you don't need to worry about keeping bottled milk sterile. If you're caught out somewhere and it's time for a feed you can simply put the baby to the breast – you don't have to hurry home with a screaming baby and make up a feed.

Although some people frown on mothers breast feeding in public, attitudes are changing at last so there is no need to be embarrassed. You can feed very discreetly if you give a little thought to what you are wearing. A button-through blouse is better than a tight fitting T-shirt, but in point of fact a loose sweat-shirt or jumper can be equally as good since you can simply tuck your baby under it with the minimum of fuss. With a loose coat or shawl strategically placed as well no one could guess that you weren't simply cuddling your baby.

Going out in the evening to friends is easy too – you can

simply take the baby with you in the carry cot and feed him if he wakes. If you feel the other guests won't appreciate you feeding in front of them, or indeed if you prefer to be on your own, quietly retire to another room, but make sure again that you have suitable clothing. Most good friends would much prefer not to isolate you and will encourage you to feed the baby in company.

If you are going out somewhere where you can't take your baby, such as the theatre, cinema or a concert, you may find that it cuts across a time when your baby is likely to wake for a feed. Try to feed your baby before you go out, but in any case it isn't going to do any harm to let your baby-sitter give the baby an occasional bottle of either formula or expressed milk (see p. 69).

There is more and more awareness of the need to provide mothers with a comfortable place to feed and change their babies in public places. Motorway service areas, railway stations and airports usually provide reasonable facilities. Shops and regular restaurants still have a long way to go, but the more parents ask for them the more notice these companies will have to take.

Going back to work

Many mothers who breast feed think that they must give up altogether if they are going back to full-time work before their babies are weaned, and this view is unfortunately a reason for some women to choose bottle feeding from the start. If your career requires you to go back to work as little as six or eight weeks after the birth, breast feeding fully during that time is still the best option for both of you (see p. 13).

It is a pity that the emphasis on paid maternity leave is given to the weeks before the birth. That is not to say that women don't need that time but that there should also be a longer period of support after the birth to enable mothers to stay at home with their babies and encourage them to breast feed for that crucial first three months (see p. 14).

In practice, most people who take maternity leave, do wait to return to work much later, especially as many companies now have more generous maternity leave provision than the statutory minimum. In most cases the babies are at least three months old and most likely six or more. In the latter case your baby will be starting to move on to solid food (see p. 112) and breast feeding may already be reduced to a couple of feeds a day. If you intend to return to work before your baby is weaned you can probably still maintain one or two breast feeds while the rest are given by bottle.

Recently it has been realized that more women need to be encouraged to come back to work and a few big companies are setting up work-place nurseries for their employees and are being further encouraged by tax incentives. This will enable some women to carry on breast feeding for longer as they can go to the nursery during lunch and other breaks to feed their babies on the premises. Again this is something that needs to be encouraged, perhaps through your trade union or staff association.

Changing from breast to bottle

Even if you do hope to maintain one or two breast feeds you still have to think ahead about introducing the bottle to your baby. The idea is to reduce your own milk supply gradually so that you do not become engorged, suffer the embarrassment of leaking breasts or, worse, blocked ducts (see p. 54). You may find that your baby resists the bottle at first, although most younger babies take to it without any problem.

■ Start planning the transition at least three weeks before you go back to work. If you are having full-time help for your baby such as a nanny or child-minder you should involve her in this transitional period right from the start so she and your baby can get to know each other.

■ Make sure you have all the equipment you need for bottle feeding and sterilizing (see p. 101-2).

■ Introduce the bottle at a feed time when you know he is usually very hungry and most receptive and when yourself are relaxed. Try mid-morning or lunch-time – keep the early morning, evening and, especially, night time for breast feeding only.

■ If you are very keen you could start with expressed breast milk (see p. 69), otherwise use the formula milk of your choice. Ask your health visitor for advice if you aren't sure. For these first 'one-off' feeds you might find it most convenient to use ready-to-feed milk.

■ If your baby won't take the bottle, try a different, softer teat and experiment with hole size. You might find that the breast fed baby takes better to the system with disposable plastic bags and softer teats (see p. 101).

■ You may also find that your baby is reluctant to take a bottle from you because he can smell your milk and knows perfectly well where your breast is. This can be rather distressing because the temptation is naturally to put him to the breast when he won't take the bottle. However, this is only going to delay things, so it might be an idea to get your partner or your helper to give the bottle until your baby is used to it.

■ Over a two-week period gradually cut out more feeds per day. Try one feed for two or three days, then two feeds for three days, and so on until you are down to perhaps two breast feeds a day, probably first thing in the morning and last thing before bed (or the night feed if he is still waking). With luck this means that your milk supply will gradually subside in line with your baby's needs.

■ If you do find that you are becoming slightly engorged between feeds, try to resist doing anything to stimulate your milk further. Don't express milk if you can help it but use cold compresses to relieve the pressure. Always make sure that you have plenty of breast pads with you. The transition period can result in an awful lot of leaking as you may find your breasts let down milk at the times you would normally be giving a breast feed. This could continue to happen to a greater or lesser extent even after you have settled down to one or two feeds only a day, or have given up altogether.

▪ When you do resume your career, you may find that your milk supply is drying up. The pressures of your working life are likely to affect lactation so it is as well to be prepared to give up even the couple of comfort feeds you are giving before very long. Equally, once your baby has taken to the bottle he may simply reject the breast since sucking from a bottle is a lot easier for him.

Brothers and sisters

When you introduce a new baby into a family where there are already other children, you may experience some jealous behaviour especially from the under fives when you are breast feeding. Your toddler may well try to climb all over you while you are feeding. Unless he is actually in danger of squashing the baby, don't push him away or he will feel very rejected. Show him what is happening and try to make him feel grown-up and special because he doesn't need to feed any more. Read him a story or watch television with him while you are feeding so that he feels part of things. When your partner is at home he can give extra time and attention to the other children.

Older children need to know that they haven't been usurped in their mother's affections just because she is breast feeding their baby brother or sister. Try to set aside time for the other children when your baby is asleep. This is hard to do in the early days when you are tired but perhaps when you are resting let them come and sit on the bed with you to draw, read or watch television.

Finding that an older child is being generally difficult about the arrival of the new baby may sometimes make a mother question whether she really ought to be breast feeding. It probably wouldn't make any difference if the baby was being bottle fed – the child would need the same amount of reassurance. On the other hand, a second child often has less attention paid to him than the first. Inevitably your time is stretched further, so breast feeding is a way of ensuring he has your more or less undivided attention at least some of the time! Breast feeding usually goes much better second or third time round. You don't have the same anxieties and apprehensions as you do with your first baby and so it is all a lot more efficient, leaving you more time for your older child.

SEVEN

Bottle feeding

Even though breast feeding is the most natural way of feeding your baby, bottle feeding may well be your preferred choice, or perhaps there are circumstances where bottle feeding is the only option (see p. 18-19). Even if you do breast feed, it may be that you need to give the odd bottle of expressed breast milk (see p. 69) or formula, or you may decide to change from breast to bottle before your baby is weaned on to solid food, perhaps because you are going back to work (see p. 95). Whatever your circumstances, it is important to know all the facts about sterilizing, making up and giving bottle feeds to your baby.

One of the biggest problems with bottle feeding is the number of 'do's and don'ts' you have to remember – which is why it really is a lot less convenient that breast feeding. It is difficult to write about bottle feeding without seeming a bit negative – 'you *must* wash your hands', 'you *shouldn't* re-use milk', 'it's *dangerous* to use too many scoops' etc. It's worth keeping this in mind if you're reading this while you are still deciding whether to breast feed or not as it might just help you to decide (see p. 22).

Equipment for bottle feeding

If you're going to bottle feed from the start you need to buy the equipment and know how to use it before you bring your baby home from hospital. In the hospital you will probably be provided with small prepacked bottles of milk, and someone else will be taking care of all the preparation, so although some hospitals do give a demonstration either at antenatal classes or on the postnatal ward, you might miss it so it's best to familiarize yourself at home. If you switch from breast to bottle, make sure you have everything you need before you start the process.

Apart from bottles, teats and sterilizing equipment, (see p. 102), you may need a couple of plastic feeding spoons, and a bottle brush and measuring jug which should be kept only for the baby's bottles and feeds.

Bottles and teats

You need enough bottles to enable you to make up several feeds at a time – at least four, and six is preferable if you are bottle feeding a newborn baby. You also need lots of teats, although you may have to experiment to find the one that best suits your baby. Bottles are now invariably made of plastic which makes them much lighter to hold. Although you can buy small bottles which only hold up to about 4 fl oz (100-125ml), these will only last you for the first three or four weeks so it is sensible to buy full size bottles right from the start.

There are two main types of bottle: the more conventional one with a rigid bottle holding the milk and a teat held in place with a screw cap, and the newer type which involves a plastic holder with disposable plastic bags for the milk which are held firmly in place by a large soft teat. This latter type has the practical advantage of not requiring a large sterilizing unit (see p. 102) because only the teats and teat covers need to be sterilized – the disposable bags are already sterile. In addition the whole system mimics breast feeding much more than a conventional bottle; there is no need to interrupt the baby's feed to allow air in as you do with a conventional bottle because the bag collapses as the milk is sucked out, and the large soft teat extends into the baby's mouth like a real nipple when he sucks.

The hole size is important with teats. The milk should drip out steadily when held upside down. If it is too small the milk comes out too slowly and the teat often gets blocked, which is frustrating for both of you. If it is too big the milk comes out too fast and may cause him to choke and splutter.

Sterilizing equipment

You need a large plastic tank in which to immerse all your baby feeding equipment to sterilize it before every feed. You can buy these in large chemists or baby care shops and departments, or you might be able to pick up a good second-hand one through your local paper or clinic. It is sensible to get one that is designed to hold your chosen type of bottle.

Whatever you choose, the tank should be large enough to take four bottles standing upright, and have a close-fitting cover to avoid anything getting into the water to contaminate it. Sterilizing solution can be bought in liquid form or in simple tablets which dissolve quickly in cold water.

It is now possible to buy a steam sterilizer which sterilizes the bottles and equipment in as little as six minutes, depending on the make. The bottles etc. no longer need to be rinsed. This system costs three to four times the amount of the ordinary plastic tank.

You need to go on sterilizing your baby's bottles and equipment for at least the first six months of life, including everything you use for solid feeding (see p. 112). If he is continuing to drink milk from a bottle it is safer to go on sterilizing until he is 12 months old.

How to sterilize

Strict attention to hygiene and sterilization of equipment is very important when you are bottle feeding as bacteria can grow all too quickly in milk, even in tiny deposits left inside the teat or within the grooves around the top of the bottle. The sort of bacterial infections that might be transmitted to your baby are very serious and may even require hospitalization so should be avoided. Sterilization techniques are given step-by-step below; it is a good idea to get into a routine and stick to it. Although the new sterilization solutions work within as little as an hour, the water should always be changed every 24 hours, so it makes sense to do the whole process at the same time every day.

■ Bottles should be washed out thoroughly after every feed with a bottle brush, and teats rinsed inside and out with salt to get rid of any milk deposits. Rinse thoroughly under running water. If you have a dishwasher, it's a good idea to wash bottle feeding equipment in it because it does get it exceptionally clean.

■ Thoroughly wash and rinse your hands.

■ Fill the sterilizing tank with the necessary amount of cold water and add sterilizing tablets or solution according to the manufacturer's instructions.

■ Stand the bottles in the solution making sure they are completely immersed and that there are no air bubbles trapped inside them. Put teats into the water upside down so that they are also completely immersed, and put anything else that you use for the baby – caps, screw tops, spoons (plastic only), and dummies – into the water, again making sure that no air bubbles are trapped inside or under them.

■ Put on the cover and leave for at least the length of time recommended by the manufacturer for sterilization to take place. Always wash and rinse your hands before removing anything from the sterilizer. Rinse the bottles etc. in cooled, freshly boiled water before using.

Sterilizing in a hurry
Although some sterilizing solutions now work very quickly, if they aren't available or if you need to sterilize a bottle and

teat in a hurry, you can always boil them. Boiling tends to discolour plastic bottles and teats but is effective. Place the items in a large pan of water and bring it to the boil, allowing them to boil on high heat and at a full boil for at least five minutes. Pour off the water and leave the items to cool inside the covered pan until they are cool enough to hold.

Formula milk

There are many brands of formula milk, most of which come in powdered form. All brands of infant formula have to conform to stringent standards of nutrition and hygiene in their manufacture, so there is little to choose between them except price. You can buy formula in concentrated liquid form, and also in cartons which are ready to put straight into the bottle without any special preparation. These latter are convenient for occasional use but are obviously much more expensive than powdered or concentrated formula. Most infant formulae are based on cow's milk (see p. 12), but there are others available based on soya or other non-cow's milk substances. These should *never* be given to your baby without consulting your doctor first.

Whichever formula you choose, always follow the manufacturer's instructions carefully when you are making up feeds. The proportion of powdered or liquid formula and boiled water will be set out clearly on the packaging, and if you are using powdered formula only use the measuring scoop provided with that particular brand. It is dangerous to make up the feed too strong; although you may be tempted or even advised by someone else to put in an extra scoop of milk – or worse still, baby cereal – 'to help him sleep longer', this is a myth. He won't sleep any longer and the extra salt that your baby's kidneys will have to deal with if the formula isn't diluted enough may cause dehydration and make him ill (see p. 12). On top of all that, he may become too fat.

Never add sugar to formula either. The sugar content is carefully controlled by the manufacturers to mimic that in breast milk and extra sugar will just make your baby fat and damage his developing teeth.

Making up feeds

Most brands of formula can now be simply made up in the bottle, rather than being made up in a jug and then transferred to bottles. This is not only more convenient but also avoids another stage during which bacteria could enter into the milk.

■ First wash your hands thoroughly and rinse them under running water.

■ Remove the bottle from the sterilizer and shake off any excess water. Rinse with cooled, freshly boiled water.

■ Following the manufacturer's instructions, fill the bottle with hand-hot, boiled water. Bottles are now marked so that you can measure in fluid ounces or millilitres.

■ Add the powdered formula one scoop at a time. Don't pack the milk down into the scoop and level each one off with a sterile knife. This will give you the exact amount required. *Only put in the recommended number of scoops for the amount of water you have put into the bottle.*

■ Put on the teat and cap. Shake the bottle vigorously to make sure all the powder has dissolved into the water. Set the bottle aside to cool down to at least blood temperature before giving it to your baby.

■ Most people make up a batch of three or four feeds at a time. Invert the teats, put the caps on, allow the milk to cool and place the extra bottles in the refrigerator until they are needed.

If you use concentrated liquid formula, it usually requires making up a whole tin in a large measuring jug and transferring it to bottles, so this type of formula does require forethought, otherwise you waste a lot of the concentrate. The

Making up a feed

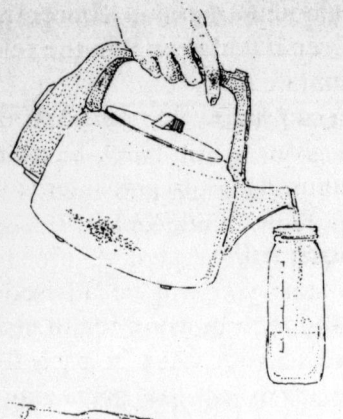

1   Fill the sterilized bottle with the right amount of boiled water. (Follow the instructions on the packet or tin.)

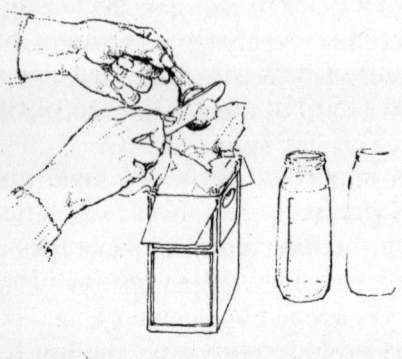

2   Insert the correct number of scoops, levelling off excess powder with a knife. Don't press it down.

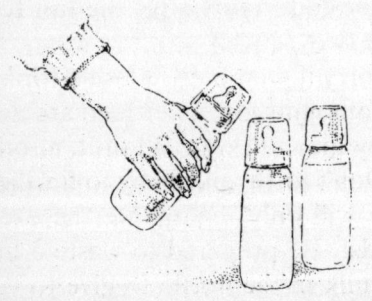

3   Cover the bottle tightly, then shake vigorously until all the powder is dissolved. Allow to cool and store in the refrigerator for up to 24 hours.

top of the can should be washed, then sterilized by pouring boiling water over it. Punch two holes with a sterilized opener. Never use a small amount of liquid concentrate, saving the rest for use later. Even if you keep it in the refrigerator it could become contaminated.

Ready-made liquid formula can simply be poured straight into the sterilized bottle and given to the baby. Don't add water and, again, don't keep unused milk to give later.

How much milk

If you bottle feed from the start you will be advised by the midwives in the hospital and then by your health visitor about how much milk to give to your baby at each feed. There will also be a guide given on the packaging of your chosen brand of formula. Normally, a newborn baby takes about 3 fl oz (85 ml) of milk at a feed, and this will gradually rise to 5-6 fl oz (150-170 ml) by the age of three months.

However, it is just as important not to be rigid about bottle feeding, as it is for breast feeding. Your baby's needs will fluctuate both during the day and over the weeks and months. Instead of forcing your baby into a routine of four-hourly feeds, simply feed him when he is hungry, just like a breast fed baby. This may be four hours after the last feed, but it might just as easily be two.

Equally, you shouldn't worry if your baby doesn't drink all the milk in the bottle. The amounts given per feed are averages – sometimes your baby may not want all of it; at other times he may want more. Don't force your baby to finish the bottle, the chances are, he will only regurgitate the excess milk all over you afterwards! Be prepared to waste a little milk. Don't keep leftover milk in the bottle to give to your baby later. Pour it away and give a fresh bottle if he is hungry again. If you make up several feeds at a time and your baby doesn't drink all of them, always throw away any milk left over after twenty-four hours and start afresh the next day.

Giving a feed

A bottle fed baby can have just as much cuddling as a breast fed baby, with the added advantage of allowing both parents to give feeds. Babies actually need the close contact of feeding, so don't be tempted to prop your baby up with a bottle by himself. This is in fact extremely dangerous as he could easily choke or breathe regurgitated milk into his lungs, or, milk might run back into the Eustachian tubes, which lead into the ear from the back of the throat, causing an ear infection. Sometimes parents of twins prop up one twin while holding the other, but this should only be done if the baby who is not being held is lying close to the parent who is feeding so that a constant watch can be kept.

There is no need to warm the bottle before you give it to the baby; many babies are quite happy to take milk straight from the refrigerator, or you could let it stand for a minute simply to take the chill off. If you want to warm it a little, simply stand the bottle in a pan of hot water for a minute or two and then shake the bottle thoroughly. Electric bottle warmers are a waste of money and can be positively dangerous if you leave a bottle warming in one too long, as it creates the perfect environment for the rapid development of dangerous bacteria. You should not warm a baby's bottle in a microwave oven as the milk will be scalding while the bottle remains cool.

If you're giving a freshly-made bottle of milk, you must let it cool down at least to blood heat before giving it to your baby. Test this by shaking a few drops onto the back of your hand or your wrist. It should not feel at all hot. It is very easy to burn a baby's mouth as the skin is much more heat-sensitive than an adult's.

■ Always wash your hands before giving a feed.

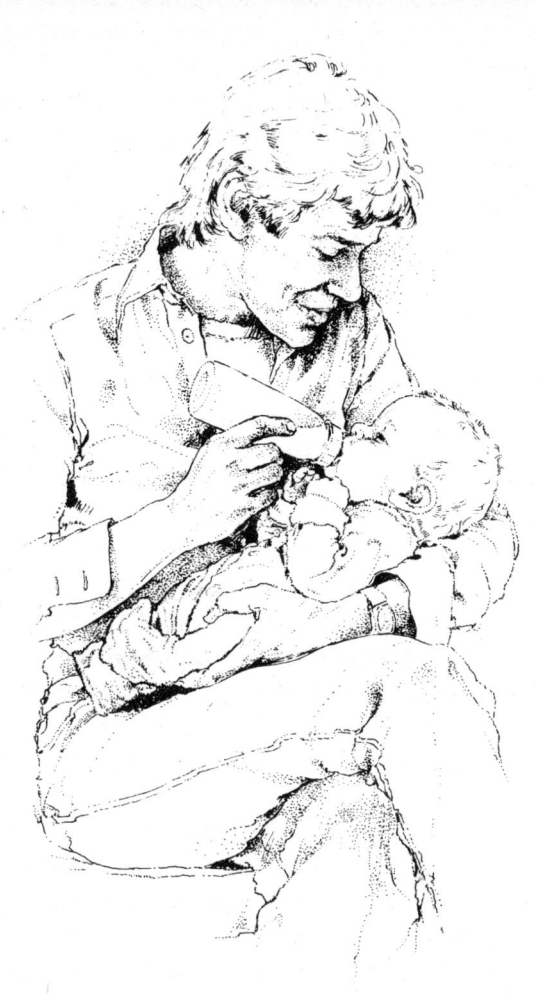

Position for giving a bottle

Cradle the baby in your arms and keep the bottle angled so that the teat is always full of milk and the baby does not swallow air.

■ Cradle your baby comfortably in your arms, propping yourself up with pillows or cushions just as you would if you were breast feeding (see p. 43) to avoid getting back ache or tired arms. Hold the bottle at a sufficient angle so that the teat is always full of milk. This ensures that the baby isn't swallowing air with the milk.

■ To encourage the small baby to suck, stroke his cheek with the teat or a finger so that he turns towards the teat and opens his mouth (see p. 36). Hold the bottle firmly so that the baby can pull against it with his suction.

■ Allow your baby to take his time. If you use a rigid bottle he'll soon learn to pause from time to time to allow air into the bottle. The temptation is to hurry him along, but a baby naturally sucks in bursts with pauses in between and it is sensible to let him develop his own rhythm.

Winding

Either in the middle or at the end of the feed, your baby may need winding. Bottle fed babies tend to swallow more air than breast fed babies and may well burp at the end of an enthusiastic feed. However, if your baby seems to be swallowing a lot of air, the hole in the teat may be too big and you should check this, perhaps changing to a smaller size for a while.

Since babies find sucking from a bottle quite easy they tend to guzzle their feeds more quickly than when breast feeding; this means that there is more likelihood of regurgitation. Make sure you have plenty of tissues or a cloth handy when winding to avoid too many stained clothes. If your baby vomits a whole feed, you should always take him to your doctor.

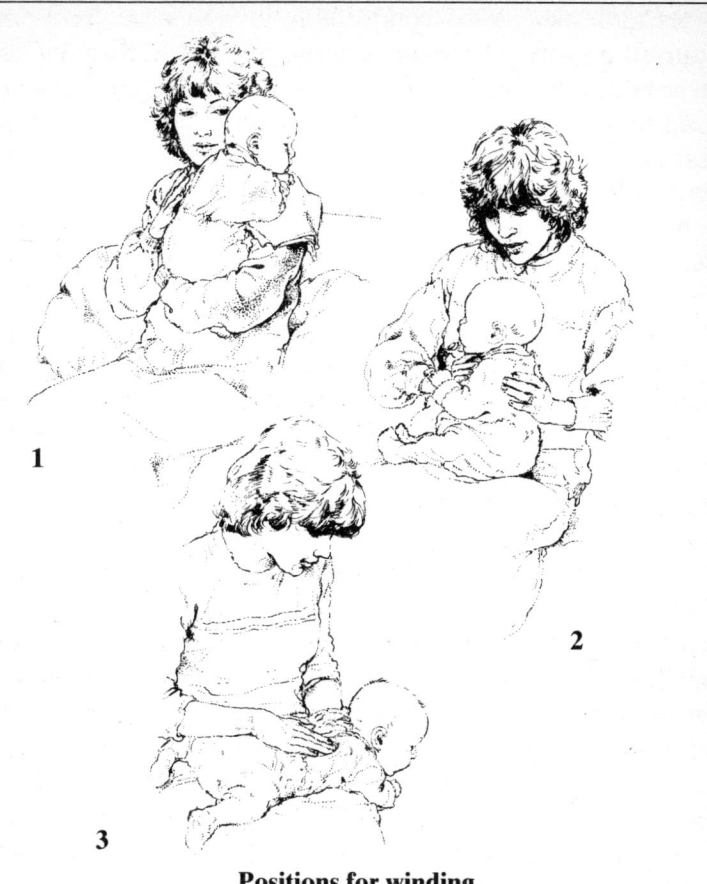

Positions for winding

1   Hold your baby over your shoulder, this often results in wind being released naturally. Have a cloth handy in case he regurgitates any milk.

2   Sit your baby on your knee, supporting his wobbly head and chest with one hand while gently rubbing his back with the other.

3   A very restless baby can often be soothed by laying him across your knees and gently massaging his back.

EIGHT

Weaning

If there is no special reason for introducing bottle feeding, such as going back to work, you can continue breast feeding for as long as you and your baby want to. However, at the age of about six months, breast milk can no longer provide all the nutritional needs of your baby and by that age your baby should be starting on a more varied diet. In practice most people introduce non-milk foods before this, and most doctors and health visitors recommend that you start at about four months, depending on your baby's weight.

Even when your baby is having three solid meals a day it still doesn't mean you have to give up breast feeding. Many mothers continue to offer the breast once or twice a day beyond their babies' first birthday, perhaps first thing in the morning or as a way of settling the baby at bedtime. By this time the 'feed' is really for comfort and pleasure and you may well find that your baby gives you up rather than the other way round at about eight or ten months. By this time he will probably be much happier with the solid food he is getting, and if you have introduced a bottle he may well prefer that to your breast, or if he has discovered his thumb he may find this a lot more handy than a breast for comfort sucking!

Many breast fed babies never drink from a bottle at all. If you continue to breast feed while you introduce solids, you can then teach your baby to drink from a cup or beaker with a feeding spout from about six months.

Introducing solid food

Although breast milk is sufficient nourishment up to about six months, you need to be a very determined mother to avoid introducing solids before then. Your baby may well start demanding more to satisfy his hunger and you could be back to three-hourly feeds. If at the age of about four months your baby is gaining weight and seems otherwise happy, but does seem to need more milk, this may be the right time to introduce solids. Check with your doctor or health visitor if you aren't sure.

Be prepared to be patient about starting your baby on solids. He is going to have to get used to the spoon and the texture of the food, and he probably won't know what to do with the first few mouthfuls and will spit them out. Baby rice mixed with a little formula or expressed breast milk is probably the best starter food. It should be very liquid and you will probably only be giving one or two tiny spoonfuls to start with.

As always, you should pay great attention to hygiene. Your baby's spoons and drinking cup (if appropriate) should be sterilized until your baby is at least six months old (see p. 102), and any bowls or other utensils you use for your baby should be thoroughly washed and rinsed, and kept separate from the rest of the family's things.

Giving solid food

■ Always wash your hands before preparing the food and giving it to your baby. Make sure the food is not too hot before you offer it. Don't add sugar; your baby will find it quite acceptable without but if he gets used to it he will find it more difficult to accept savoury foods later. Refined sugar is bad for babies; it makes them fat and encourages tooth decay even before the first teeth have come through. It is also important not to add salt to the baby's food because extra salt can stress immature kidneys.

■ If you are giving ready-prepared baby food there is no real reason to heat it as your baby won't know whether it tastes better hot or cold. *Never* heat a baby's food in a microwave oven.

■ When you start solids, choose a time when your baby is alert and happy, and you have the peace and quiet to concentrate. Like changing from breast to bottle, this is best done during the day rather than first thing in the morning when he is very hungry or last thing at night when you want him to settle down to sleep after the feed. You could fit it in to the middle of a feed, perhaps offering one breast to satisfy his immediate hunger, and then putting him to the other breast when he has tried some solids.

■ Hold your baby on your knee or harness him into his baby chair. A rigid baby chair is better than a bouncing cradle as there is less likelihood of him bouncing the spoon out of your hand, but you shouldn't put him in a regular high chair until he can sit up unaided. Never put your baby in his bouncing cradle on a table or work top as he may easily 'bounce' it off.

■ Make sure he has a large bib or better still a tea-towel or muslin nappy covering his clothes. Feeding is a messy business. Protect your own clothes with an apron too!

■ Put a little food on the tip of the spoon and gently tickle his upper lip with it to persuade him to open his mouth. Don't try and force his mouth open; he'll only turn his head away and the food will go everywhere at which point he may become frightened or confused which will make the job even harder.

■ Once he's opened his mouth let him suck the food off the end of the spoon. You may be highly amused by the faces he makes as he experiences this new sensation – he may spit the food out or forget to swallow so that it just dribbles out again. But he'll soon get the idea.

■ Two or three spoonfuls at any one feed is quite enough

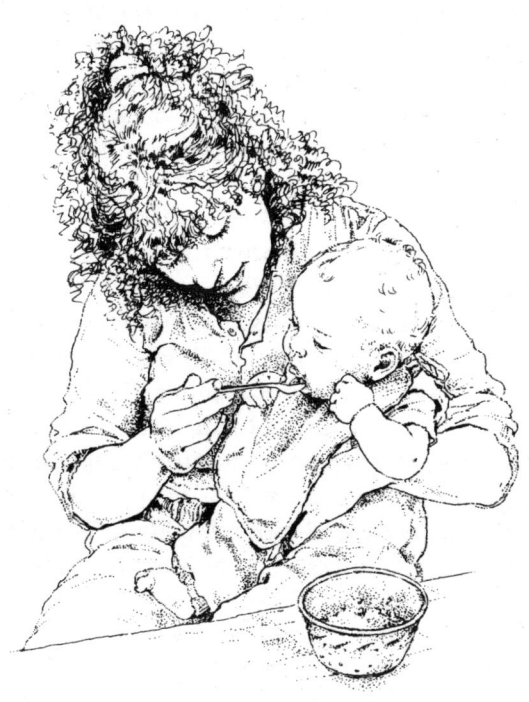

How to introduce solids

Sit at a table holding your baby firmly on your lap. With a little food on the tip of the spoon, stroke his upper lip and let him suck the food off it.

for the first few tries. This provides a really significant increase in calories compared with milk feeds, and even the blandest baby rice requires much harder work from your baby's digestive system so he needs time to get used to it.

■ You can gradually increase the amounts, and also introduce new tastes and types of food as the days pass. Only introduce one new food at a time, and be prepared for rejections. If your baby decides he doesn't like the taste of puréed potato this week, go back to something you know he does like and re-introduce the potatoes a few days later.

Your baby's diet

While you are still mainly breast feeding you don't have to worry too much about maintaining a balanced diet. Breast milk provides all the nourishment that your baby needs and the solids are supplementary. Once your baby is used to taking food from the spoon provide as wide a variety of tastes as you can as he will be pretty undiscriminating about food at this stage.

Although pre-packaged baby foods are perfectly acceptable, especially the powdered variety to which you simply have to add boiled water, freshly cooked foods are better and cheaper in the long run. Puréed vegetables can be served by themselves or with meat or fish stock added, and you can also use dried vegetables such as lentils or beans. Offer cooked, puréed fruit (add a little sugar or honey to very tart fruits like cooking apples), although you may find that citrus or soft fruits can result in rather loose stools at first.

Always cook the food thoroughly to start with, then sieve or blend it into a smooth paste. Add more boiled water, stock or milk to thin it if it is too stiff. If you make too much for one meal, freeze the rest in small batches. The ice-tray is a useful container for this. However, don't use a microwave oven to defrost or warm up your baby's food as you cannot be sure that it has killed off all bacteria.

If you are reheating food make sure that it is properly cooked through – it takes at least ten minutes boiling to kill off harmful bacteria. Always throw away leftover foods from the baby's bowl; if you have food left over in a jar or tin, transfer it into a clean bowl and store it covered in the refrigerator for not more than twenty-four hours. If you haven't used it by then throw it away. This may seem a waste but it is better than risking contamination with bacteria.

It is best to avoid eggs until your baby is older, although you could blend in hard-boiled egg with mashed potato or cheese sauce. It is also best to use a hard cheese such as cheddar or Swiss cheese. By the time your baby is about six months old you will probably find that he is eating solid food three times a day, very much as the rest of the family. You should therefore aim to balance his diet with vegetables, fruit, dairy produce and meat and fish if you want. The more different types of food he eats at this age the less likely he is to be faddy about foods later.

A typical day's nourishment at six to eight months might consist of an early morning breast feed at 6.30 or 7 a.m., followed by breakfast of baby cereal and perhaps juice from a cup at 9 o'clock. Depending on your baby's sleep pattern, you might be giving him lunch at twelve, consisting of puréed meat or fish and a vegetable, perhaps followed by mashed banana and plain yoghurt, with juice in a cup. Lunchtime is very often the first milk feed to be dropped altogether, whether you are feeding by breast or bottle. Then at tea-time your baby may have a drink, either from the cup or breast, followed by a meal consisting of puréed cauliflower cheese or something similar. Then there will probably be another full breast feed after his bath and before you settle him for the night. A significant number of babies of this age will still be waking at some point in the night and want to feed again.

Drinking from a cup

You can introduce a cup to your baby from about six months. Nowadays most people use the special training beakers with spouts. These cups have the benefit of avoiding too many spills and babies generally start by sucking the liquid out of them. Other parents introduce an ordinary cup straight away and it may surprise you how quickly babies learn to drink from a cup quite efficiently without too many spills. Either way, there really isn't any necessity to give drinks in a bottle if you are continuing to breast feed.

Provide unsweetened fruit juice or plain boiled water to drink. It's probably wise to dilute fruit juices with water to start with as they are quite acidic. Try to avoid sweet baby drinks or squashes as they are very sugary and bad for developing teeth. There shouldn't be any need to give milk until you have stopped breast feeding altogether. You can provide extra milk and calcium-rich foods if you want with yoghurt and cheese, and use ordinary cow's milk for cereals.

Pasteurized milk from your milkman is quite suitable for your baby from about six months of age, and it probably isn't necessary to boil it as long as it is fresh and has been kept in the refrigerator. Special formula milk for older babies is a waste of money; don't bother with it.

Self-feeding

Your baby may show signs of wanting to feed himself from as early as eight months. By this time he'll be sitting in a high chair (make sure there is a harness for him) and can sometimes join you for family meals. Even before his teeth break through he'll be starting to chew so you can begin to offer hard foods like pieces of apple and raw carrot to hold and gnaw himself. Don't leave him alone with finger foods however just in case a small piece breaks off and he chokes.

When he starts trying to grab the spoon you'll know he's ready to start feeding himself. This can be time consuming and frustrating for the busy parent but it's worth persevering because it will will save you a lot of time in the long run when he can feed himself and you'll be helping him develop his manual skills. Give him a spoon and have one of your own so you can pop mouthfuls in while he is desperately trying to do it himself.

This stage can be incredibly messy. If this bothers you, lay plastic sheeting under his chair to catch the worst of the bits. It can be particularly irritating if he starts refusing food altogether or throwing the bowl onto the floor. Try to be patient and never force your baby to eat when he really doesn't want to. He may not be very hungry, or perhaps the taste or texture of the food is unfamiliar. Give him another breast feed and try again later when you are both calmer.

Breast feeding the older baby
Occasionally mothers continue to nurse their older babies and toddlers till they are two years or even older. A young child who is still nursing at this age is not getting much nourishment, he is doing it for comfort, just as another child might suck her thumb or drink from a bottle.

Continuing to breast feed for this long is entirely up to you. You need to decide whether you are happy to allow your child to be dependent on your body in this way. If it suits you and your child, that's fine, but some women have found it a mixed blessing, since their young children tend to think of their mothers' breasts as their property to be nursed whenever they want. It is worth bearing in mind that by eighteen months or two years, your toddler will be talking and will certainly have found a word for his favourite comforter. It can be embarrassing when your toddler starts shouting in the supermarket for his 'titty' or 'booby' or whatever term he has chosen for it. In the end, using the breast as a comforter isn't going to do any harm, but it is harder to break the habit than hiding the bottle or dummy.

NINE

Looking after your breasts

Once you have breast fed one baby, you will find it easy to breast feed any subsequent babies. Only very rarely does a mother find that she cannot breast feed again; it is usually because of unforeseen illness requiring medication which would be bad for the baby. After you have finished feeding your first baby, you will notice that your breasts have changed slightly in appearance. Your nipples and areola will be a bit darker than before you were pregnant and your breasts may well be smaller (see p. 49) or be slightly less uplifted as the ligaments that support the breasts may be less taut.

While you are pregnant and feeding your baby, it is natural that you should be particularly aware of your breasts and the changes that are taking place in them, just as you arc with all the reproductive organs in your body. You will find that the doctors and midwives who are caring for you will always include breast examination in their general assessment of your health. When breast feeding is finished most women ignore their breasts until another pregnancy brings them into focus again.

However, it is sensible to check your breasts from time to time as a way of preventing problems arising later. Most breast lumps are found by women themselves, or sometimes their partners, and not by doctors during routine examinations. There has been quite a lot of publicity recently about setting up mass screening for breast problems, but in point of fact this screening is mainly targeted at women over the age of fifty-five, when most cases of breast cancer occur. Your doctor may well examine your breasts routinely when you go for some other treatment, such as problems with menstruation, for family planning advice or for a cervical smear test. At best this is only going to be once a year, and probably much more sporadically, so it is sensible to make a habit of examining your own breasts once a month, and no less than every three months.

If you don't already do this, you needn't feel too guilty. At least you know that there are plenty of women like you. It is sometimes hard to find the time, privacy or inclination to examine your own breasts thoroughly and quite a lot of women put off examining their breasts because they are frightened of actually finding something amiss. It is important to realize however that there are plenty of conditions that cause breast lumps which have nothing to do with cancer, and if a cancerous lump is discovered, it can be treated extremely effectively. It is also worth remembering that if you have had children and have breast fed them, statistically you have a lower risk of breast cancer than a childless woman.

Breast self-examination

When you examine your breasts you will be looking for lumps of tissue that feel completely separate or 'discrete', to use the medical term, rather than generalized lumpiness or 'stringiness'. Very many women experience breast tenderness, swelling and lumpiness in the two weeks before menstruation; this is because the hormones which control the reproductive cycle affect all parts of the body associated with reproduction and as has been said earlier, the breasts and breast feeding are an integral part of that process (see p. 24). The lumpiness is caused by temporary enlargement of the glandular tissue in the breast and is usually felt towards the outer edges of the breasts. It is very different from the lumps associated with other breast conditions.

This means it is better to get into the habit of examining your breasts in the week after your period has finished. Any swelling associated with menstruation will have subsided and it will be less confusing. When you decide to examine your breasts, make sure you have five minutes to yourself in a warm room or bathroom with a large mirror in which you can see yourself from the waist up.

▪ First of all stand in front of the mirror with your arms by your sides and look at your breasts. Most people's breasts are slightly different shapes; but what you are looking for here is an obvious protrusion in the outline, or, just as important, a depression or puffiness in the skin.

▪ Then, raise your arms above your head and look at your breasts again, particularly the underside.

▪ Finally, lean forward and look at your breasts with the weight pulling them down to enable you to see the upper part and sides.

▪ When you have completed these procedures lie down comfortably on the bed or in the bath. Put one arm up behind your head, and feel the breast on that side with the other hand. Always use the flat part of your middle three fingers. Gently massage in a circular motion the top, sides and underside of your breast to see if there is anything different. Feel in your armpit for enlarged lymph nodes by sliding your hand from the highest point you can reach down through your armpit on to your ribs. Then repeat the whole process on the other breast and armpit.

▪ If your breasts are very full, use two hands to examine them. Support the top with one hand while you examine the under side with the other and vice versa.

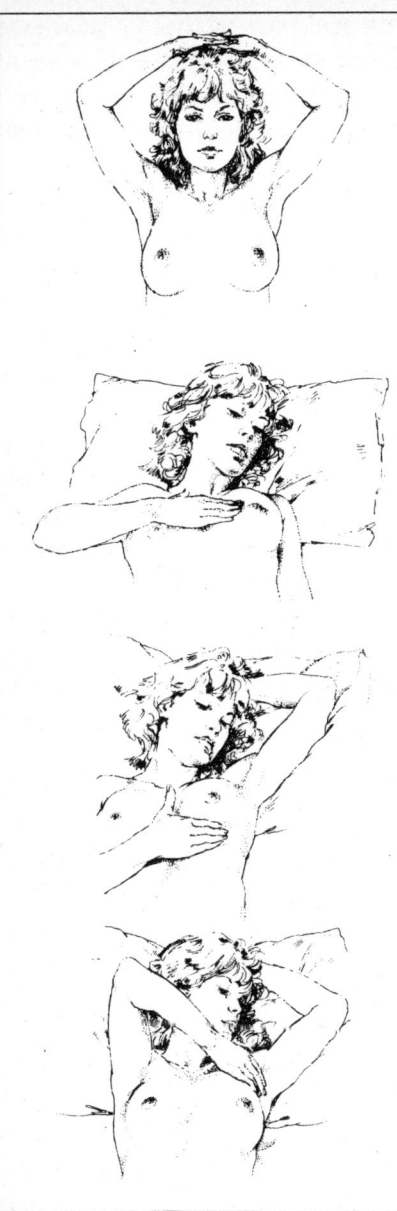

Breast examination

1   Stand in front of a mirror, raise both arms above your head and turn from side to side to look for unusual irregularities in the outline of your breasts.

2   Lie flat, and with your fingers straight and flat, feel the top half of your breast for lumps with the opposite hand, moving in a circular, clockwise motion. Do not press too hard, and leave the arm not in use straight by your side.

3   Feel the lower half of your breast in the same way, but with the free arm behind your head.

4   Follow this manoeuvre by feeling for lumps in the tissue leading up to the armpit. Feel right into the armpit as well. Repeat the whole process with the other breast.

What to report to your doctor

If you are at all worried about your breasts, always go to your family doctor for a quick check. He or she can reassure you straight away if there is nothing to worry about. Remember once again that by no means all lumps are malignant (cancerous), and even if you are found to have a malignant lump it can be treated, which nowadays almost certainly means that you will not have to have your whole breast removed.

See your doctor immediately in the following situations.

■ If you find a lump don't wait to see if it goes away.

■ If you experience localized pain, particularly if it is associated with a lump. Think about whether you are due for a period, or whether you have been doing any unaccustomed activity which might actually be causing a feeling of stiffness in your pectoral muscles underneath the breast. Pain is rarely present in discrete cancerous lumps.

■ If there is a patch of discoloured skin or skin dimpled like orange peel, particularly if the area is slightly depressed or pulled inward. This dimpled effect is particularly obvious when the arms are raised above the head.

■ If your nipple seems to be inverted or pulled inwards, when it never has been before.

■ If there is any form of discharge from the nipple at a time when you are neither pregnant or lactating.

Useful addresses

When writing for information please enclose a stamped addressed envelope. All addresses and telephone numbers are correct at the time of going to press.

The National Childbirth Trust (NCT)
Alexandra House
Oldham Terrace
London W3 6NH
081-992 6762
Antenatal classes and postnatal support

La Leche League
BCM 3424
London WC1N 3XX
071-242 1278
Breast feeding advice and support

Association of Breastfeeding Mothers
26 Holmshaw Close
London SE26 4TH
081-778 4769
Postnatal support

The Maternity Alliance
15 Britannia Street
London WC1X 9JP
071-837 1265
Campaigns for improvements in rights and services for parents and babies

NIPPERS (National Information for Parents of
Prematures)
c/o Perinatal Research Unit
St Mary's Hospital
Praed Street
London W2 1NY
071-725 1487
Information on education, resources and support

National Caesarean Support Association
72 Perry Rise
London SE23 3QL
081-699 8399

CLAPA (Cleft Lip and Palate Association)
Speech Therapy Department
Hospital for Sick Children
Great Ormond Street
London WC1N 3JH
071-405 9200
Information and advisory service

Contact a Family
16 Strutton Ground
London SW1P 2HP
071-222 2695
*Brings together families with handicapped children for
mutual support also acts as an information centre*

In Touch
10 Norman Road
Sale
Cheshire M33 3DF
061-962 4441

Voluntary Council for the Handicapped Child
National Children's Bureau
8 Wakley Street
London EC1V 7QE
071-278 9441
Information and advisory service

The Stillbirth and Neonatal Death Society (SANDS)
28 Portland Place
London W1N 4DE
071-436 5881
Support on an individual or group basis

CRY-SIS
B.M. Cry-sis
London WC1N 3XX
071-404 5011
Support group for parents of crying babies

National Council for One-Parent Families
255 Kentish Town Road
London NW5 2LX
071-267 1361
Information leaflets and advice

Association for Postnatal Illness
7 Gowan Avenue
Fulham
London SW6 6RH
071-731 4867
Offers support, mainly by telephone